Superficial Fungal Infections of the Skin

Superficial Fungal Infections of the Skin

Second Edition

Authors

Archana Singal MD FAMS
Director Professor and Head
Department of Dermatology and STD
University College of Medical Sciences and GTB Hospital
New Delhi, India

Chander Grover MD DNB MNAMS
Director Professor
Department of Dermatology and STD
University College of Medical Sciences and GTB Hospital
New Delhi, India

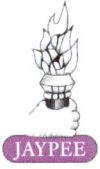

JAYPEE BROTHERS MEDICAL PUBLISHERS
The Health Sciences Publisher
New Delhi | London

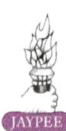 **Jaypee Brothers Medical Publishers (P) Ltd**

Headquarters
EMCA House
23/23-B, Ansari Road, Daryaganj
New Delhi 110 002, India
Landline: +91-11-23272143,
+91-11-23272703, +91-11-23282021
+91-11-23245672
E-mail: jaypee@jaypeebrothers.com

Corporate Office
Jaypee Brothers Medical Publishers (P) Ltd.
4838/24, Ansari Road, Daryaganj
New Delhi 110 002, India
Phone: +91-11-43574357
Fax: +91-11-43574314
E-mail: jaypee@jaypeebrothers.com

Overseas Office
JP Medical Ltd.
83, Victoria Street, London
SW1H 0HW (UK)
Phone: +44-20 3170 8910
Fax: +44(0)20 3008 6180
E-mail: info@jpmedpub.com

EU GPSR Authorised Representative
LOGOS EUROPE, 9 rue Nicolas Poussin
17000, LA ROCHELLE, France
Phone: +33 (0) 6 67 93 73 78
Email: Contact@logos europe.eu

Website: www.jaypeebrothers.com
Website: www.jaypeedigital.com

© 2024, Jaypee Brothers Medical Publishers

The views and opinions expressed in this book are solely those of the original contributor(s)/author(s) and do not necessarily represent those of editor(s) or publisher of the book.

All rights reserved. No part of this publication may be reproduced, stored or transmitted in any form or by any means, electronic, mechanical, photocopying, recording or otherwise, without the prior permission in writing of the publishers.

All brand names and product names used in this book are trade names, service marks, trademarks or registered trademarks of their respective owners. The publisher is not associated with any product or vendor mentioned in this book.

Medical knowledge and practice change constantly. This book is designed to provide accurate, authoritative information about the subject matter in question. However, readers are advised to check the most current information available on procedures included and check information from the manufacturer of each product to be administered, to verify the recommended dose, formula, method and duration of administration, adverse effects and contraindications. It is the responsibility of the practitioner to take all appropriate safety precautions. Neither the publisher nor the author(s)/editor(s) assume any liability for any injury and/or damage to persons or property arising from or related to use of material in this book.

This book is sold on the understanding that the publisher is not engaged in providing professional medical services. If such advice or services are required, the services of a competent medical professional should be sought.

Every effort has been made where necessary to contact holders of copyright to obtain permission to reproduce copyright material. If any have been inadvertently overlooked, the publisher will be pleased to make the necessary arrangements at the first opportunity.

Inquiries for bulk sales may be solicited at: jaypee@jaypeebrothers.com

Superficial Fungal Infections of the Skin / ***Archana Singal, Chander Grover***

First Edition: 2019
Second Edition: **2024**
ISBN: 978-93-5696-442-6

Preface to the Second Edition

Infections form the bulk of dermatology outpatients, especially in India. Of these, superficial fungal infections have always been a major component. The unprecedented surge in the incidence and prevalence of superficial dermatophytosis in the past one decade has brought it in the focus area of intense research activities. Significant changes have been observed and documented pertaining to their epidemiology, clinical presentations, and therapeutic interventions. The changing face of superficial fungal infections also leads to difficulties in diagnosis. However, we have an additional improved diagnostic technique available, i.e., using a dermatoscope that can facilitate diagnosis in such cases. This so-called epidemic of dermatophytosis is largely fueled by the spread of multidrug-resistant *Trichophyton* species which is supposedly an outcome of injudicious use of antifungal drugs and steroid abuse. The situation can be dealt with an informed and judicious use of oral and topical antifungal agents and avoidance of steroids. Both these aspects require major efforts in educating medical professionals, pharmacists, and patients alike.

With limited drugs in the antifungal armamentarium, it is a daunting task to manage superficial fungal infections, which were earlier considered easy-to-treat infections. In addition, tropical climate with high temperature and humidity, overcrowding, use of occlusive clothing, and sharing facilitate the initiation and propagation of superficial fungal infections in the families. Rampant steroid abuse and misuse by medical professionals, pharmacists, and the patients have led to this unfortunate scenario. Till date, many irrational and harmful fixed-drug combinations of potent steroid molecules with antifungal, antibiotic, and antiparasitic molecules are available for topical use. Over-the-counter availability and unrestricted access to the general public have made the matter worse. In addition, prevalent comorbidities like diabetes mellitus or other causes of immunosuppression often result in extensive, recalcitrant fungal infections.

The only remedial measure is to disseminate correct information and to educate the treating physicians. We attempted to do it through the first edition, which was very well received. This prompted the publication of the second edition. The second edition of this book, "*Superficial Fungal Infections of the Skin*", is our sincere and earnest effort to educate medical health professionals, who regularly encounter such patients in their practice. The chapters deal extensively with the causative factors of recalcitrant tinea as well as its changing and atypical clinical presentations. A devoted chapter on dermoscopy has been added demonstrating the unique features useful in diagnosis of skin, hair, and nail infections. The section on therapy provides details regarding not only the treatment schedules but also the general instruction to be given to the patients to comprehensively address the problem. A large number of clinical pictures have been added in this edition, to help maintain the interest in the subject and ensure lucidity of text.

We welcome constructive thoughts and suggestions, which can help us improve the content further, so that the book serves its purpose well.

Archana Singal
Chander Grover

Preface to the First Edition

Infections continue to contribute significantly to morbidity and mortality worldwide, particularly in the developing world. Since last 6–7 years, there has been an unprecedented and significant change in the epidemiology, clinical features and therapeutic intervention of Superficial Dermatophytosis. Latter has gained the proportion of an epidemic. With limited drugs in the antifungal armamentarium, it is a daunting task to treat otherwise easy, superficial fungal infections. In addition to the suitable climatic conditions of tropical countries like India such as high temperature, humidity and overcrowding required for the initiation and propagation of fungal infections, steroid abuse/misuse for each and every skin lesion/blemishes by non-dermatologist is to be blamed for this change. It is unfortunate that many irrational and harmful fixed drug combinations of potent steroid molecule with antifungal, antibiotic, antiparasitic molecules are available for topical use. An initial transitory response due to anti-inflammatory property of steroid is followed by havoc of difficult to treat fungal/tinea infections. In addition, prevalent comorbidities like diabetes mellitus result in extensive fungal infections. In such a scenario, it is very relevant to have a dedicated manual addressing the problem of fungal infections that are difficult to identify, diagnose and treat. This book has concise information about the atypical presentation in different age groups, latest diagnostic techniques including office based procedures like dermatoscopy. A large number of clinical pictures maintains the interest in the subject and lucidity. This book promises to be an anthology of superficial fungal infections and their management from a dermatological perspective.

We welcome readers' criticism and suggestions, which will help us improve and refine subsequent publications.

Archana Singal
Chander Grover

Acknowledgments

We wish to acknowledge the encouragement we received from our readers of our previous books on Dermatologic Infections! This book contains concise, super-relevant information to efficiently diagnose and appropriately manage superficial dermatophytosis. A large number of clinical photographs enhance its visual appeal and maintain readers' interest.

We express our immense gratitude towards our patients who have taught us so much over the years and enabled us to take on the new diagnostic and therapeutic challenges. No amount of written material or internet searches can yield the wealth of information or the gift of satisfaction we receive by interacting and treating them.

We thank our department and institution for the academic freedom and necessary support and our students for constantly inspiring us to learn more and more. We also thank our authors Dr Hema Jerajani and Dr Saurabh Jindal for their contribution to the chapter on 'Normal Flora' and Dr Suruchi Bhasin for contribution to the chapter on 'Superficial Fungal Infections', both in our earlier book 'Comprehensive approach to Infections in Dermatology'.

We extend our sincere thanks to Shri Jitendar P Vij (Group Chairman), Mr Ankit Vij (Managing Director), Ms Chetna Malhotra (Senior Director—Professional Publishing, Marketing and Business Development), Mr Akhilesh Saxena (Publishing Coordinator), and all the other team members of M/s Jaypee Brothers Medical Publishers (P) Ltd, New Delhi, India, for trusting and supporting us in the publication of this book.

Last but not least, we wish to thank our families and friends for their unconditional and constant emotional support and love.

Archana Singal
Chander Grover

Contents

SECTION 1: NORMAL FLORA

1. Normal Flora of Skin   3
2. Normal Oral Flora   12
3. Factors Affecting the Skin Flora   13
4. Skin Flora in Disease   16

SECTION 2: DERMATOPHYTOSIS

5. Epidemiology and Etiology of Dermatophytosis in India   23
6. Pathogenesis of Dermatophytosis   25
7. Dermatophytosis of Skin   29
8. Recalcitrant Dermatophytosis   42
9. Tinea Capitis   61
10. Onychomycosis   66

SECTION 3: DIAGNOSIS OF DERMATOPHYTOSIS

11. Dermatoscopy (Skin, Hair, and Nail) and Bedside Diagnosis of Dermatophytosis   77
12. Laboratory Diagnosis   90

SECTION 4: TREATMENT OF DERMATOPHYTOSIS

13. General Measures   99
14. Topical Therapy   100
15. Systemic Treatment   106
16. Systemic Treatment in Special Populations   111

SECTION 5: OTHER SUPERFICIAL FUNGAL INFECTIONS

17. Candidiasis or Candidosis	115
18. Pityriasis Versicolor	131
19. Tinea Nigra Palmaris	136
20. Piedra or Trichomycosis Nodularis	138
Bibliography	141
Index	145

SECTION 1

Normal Flora

Chapter 1:   Normal Flora of Skin
Chapter 2:   Normal Oral Flora
Chapter 3:   Factors Affecting the Skin Flora
Chapter 4:   Skin Flora in Disease

CHAPTER 1

Normal Flora of Skin

INTRODUCTION

Human skin is in fact a habitat, constantly hosting an array of microbes. The surface of the skin has defense mechanisms helping it desist colonization, to prevent entry of potential pathogens. Nevertheless, complex communities of bacteria, fungi, and viruses thrive on our skin. A newborn delivered by cesarean section is sterile but soon acquires its own resident flora within the first few minutes of life. Initially, it consists of homogenous microbe types over the entire skin. However, with increasing environmental exposure and development of distinct moisture, temperature, and glandular characteristics, individual skin habitats start arising, with a heterogeneous distribution of organisms. The mixture of organisms regularly found at any anatomical site is referred to as the normal flora, more appropriately as the "microbiome".

An estimated 1 million bacteria, with hundreds of distinct species, inhabit each square centimeter of our skin. A thorough knowledge of the normal skin flora thus equips a clinician to predict the likely causative organism in disease states and helps him focus on preservation of the cutaneous flora to prevent infections.

MICROBIAL SKIN FLORA

Studies have shown that the vast majority of skin bacteria fall into four phyla: Actinobacteria, Firmicutes, *Bacteroides*, and Proteobacteria. However, within these phyla exist thousands of distinct species **(Fig. 1)**. As organisms prefer designated environmental conditions, specific areas

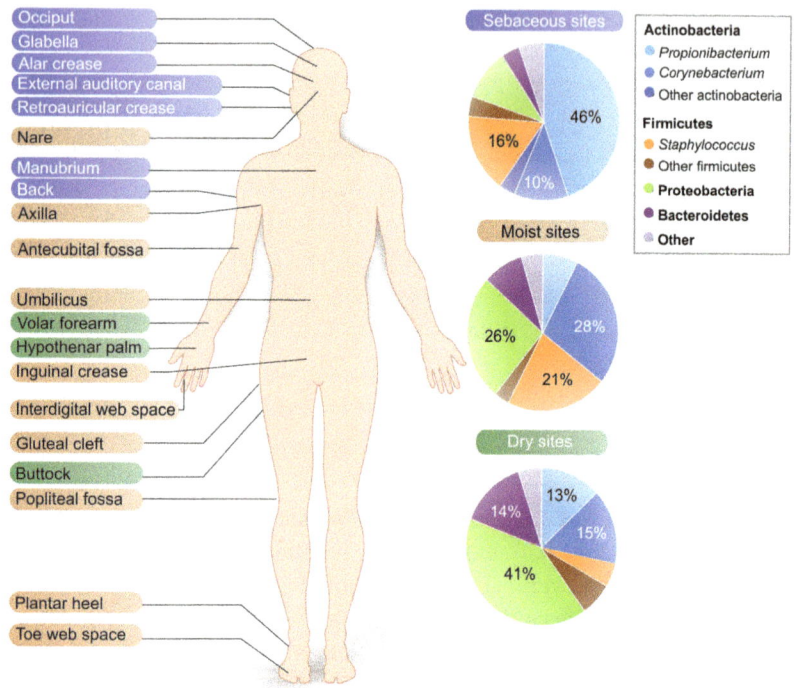

Fig. 1: Microbiome composition on normal-appearing human skin. Sebaceous (blue text), moist (orange text), and dry (green text) habitats are labeled anatomically. Microbial composition differs between habitats (pie charts at right).

Four major phyla are shown: Actinobacteria, firmicutes, proteobacteria, and bacteroidetes. Within these phyla, three most abundant genera are also shown: *Propionibacterium*, *Corynebacterium*, and *Staphylococcus*.

Source: Chen YE, Tsao H. The skin microbiome: current perspectives and future challenges. J Am Acad Dermatol. 2013;69(1):143-55.

on the human skin harbor specific flora. For instance, *Propionibacterium* species dominates sebaceous areas (such as the forehead, retroauricular crease, and back), whereas *Staphylococcus* and *Corynebacterium* species dominate moist areas (such as the axillae).

Consistent with this idea of ecological niches, it has been reported that transplanting microbes from one habitat to another (such as from the tongue to the forehead) causes only a transient presence of tongue microbiota on the forehead with eventual return to the forehead microbiome.

The existence of skin flora of three types has been proposed. These include the following:
1. *Resident flora/commensals*: This represents the first group due to its compact attachment to the skin surface. Stratum corneum and upper epidermis are the common sites for resident flora. It produces antimicrobial peptides (AMPs), which decrease the survival of pathogens on healthy human skin by two to three log fold. Sometimes, as the skin milieu gets altered or under special circumstances including immunosuppression, in-dwelling catheters, etc., the resident microflora can become pathogenic and cause infections. The organisms which are commonly part of resident flora of human skin include *Staphylococcaceae, Micrococcaceae* (earlier included staphylococci), *Peptococcus, Micrococcus*, Coryneform organisms, *Brevibacterium, Propionibacterium, Acinetobacter*, and *Pityrosporum*.
2. *Transient flora*: This represents the second group of microbes. They are called "transient" due to their free, unattached character. This group is more prevalent on the exposed skin surfaces.
3. *Temporary flora*: A third group of organisms named temporary flora has been identified of late. It colonizes the skin in a minority of individuals. These organisms need a combination of host and environmental factors to establish themselves. They also disappear under adverse conditions. For example, a physician who is not using adequate universal precautions and is exposed to infective organisms during wound dressing is likely to carry such flora. The organisms will stay until he/she is exposed and then gradually disappear from the skin.

The organisms which have been found to colonize human skin can be classified as follows.

Bacterial Flora

Bacteria comprise the largest group of colonizing microbes in human skin. The important phyla of bacteria, residing on human skin, have been listed above **(Fig. 1)**. Gram-positive cocci were earlier members of the family *Micrococcaceae*. However, it has now been redefined and the genera have been rearranged in three different families including *Staphylococcaceae*, redefined *Micrococcaceae*, and newly defined *Dermacoccaceae*. Few of the more relevant organisms are discussed below.

Family: Staphylococcaceae

Coagulase-negative staphylococci are the most frequently found resident flora of human skin. At least 18 different species of staphylococci have been isolated from normal skin; the primary residents are *Staphylococcus epidermidis, Staphylococcus hominis, Staphylococcus haemolyticus, Staphylococcus capitis, Staphylococcus warneri, Staphylococcus saprophyticus* (most common in the perineum), *Staphylococcus cohnii, Staphylococcus xylosus,* and *Staphylococcus simulans.* Of these, *S. epidermidis* and *S. hominis* are the species recovered most frequently.

Staphylococcus epidermidis colonizes the upper part of the body preferentially and constitutes more than 50% of the resident staphylococci of human skin. The forehead and the antecubital fossae carry *Staphylococcus saccharolyticus* in 20% of adults.

Staphylococcus aureus colonization is not very common on human skin, as it exhibits a great degree of natural resistance. Hence, apart from intertriginous areas and the perineum (where it touches 20% of the total flora), it is rare to find it colonizing human skin. *S. aureus* carriage is the most clinically relevant in the anterior nares with 20–40% of adults being nasal carriers. This carriage is even more common in diabetic patients, patients on hemodialysis, and those with psoriasis and atopy, thus leading to a risk of recurrent pyoderma. Addressing this common carriage site often leads to resolution of pyoderma.

Family: Micrococcaceae

Micrococci are less frequently present than staphylococci. Nevertheless, at least eight different *Micrococcus* species have been identified from human skin. In order of prevalence, these include *Micrococcus luteus, Micrococcus varians, Micrococcus lylae, Micrococcus nishinomiyaensis, Micrococcus kristinae, Micrococcus roseus, Micrococcus sedentarius,* and *Micrococcus aggies.*

Coryneform Organisms

The organisms of the genus *Corynebacterium* are classically found in the intertriginous areas. They are known as *Corynebacterium lipophilicus. Corynebacterium minutissimum,* once thought to be a single organism distinguished by its ability to produce porphyrin, is now known to be a complex organism of as many as eight different species.

Cutibacteria

Cutibacterium (formerly known as *Propionibacterium*) species are nonsporulating, gram-positive anaerobic bacilli. These are considered skin commensals and are usually nonpathogenic. They are common contaminants of blood and body fluid cultures. Cutibacteria are slow-growing, needing at least 6 days for growth in culture. They are normal residents of hair follicles and sebaceous glands, being the most prevalent anaerobes amongst the normal flora. They are also known as anaerobic coryneforms. They are divided into three species: *Cutibacterium acnes*, *Cutibacterium granulosum*, and *Cutibacterium avidum*.

Cutibacterium species are best studied because of their association with acne; however, they can also cause other infections, including endocarditis, postoperative shoulder infections, and neurosurgical shunt infections.

Cutibacterium acnes is a transient flora of neonatal skin, while true colonization starts near puberty. It thrives in the lipid-rich microenvironment of hair follicles, with highest counts on the face and upper thorax. It produces inflammatory mediators involved in the pathogenesis of acne papules, pustules, and nodulocystic lesions.

Cutibacterium granulosum colonizes the same areas, but its counts are one hundredth those of *C. acnes*. Both *C. acnes* and *C. granulosum* may be isolated from the gastrointestinal tract as well.

Cutibacterium avidum is found in the axillae (moist intertriginous areas) rather than on exposed areas. Its numbers also increase with the onset of puberty.

Gram-negative Rods

They constitute only transient flora of human skin. Due to their high requirement of moisture for propagation and survival, desiccation inhibits their growth while intertriginous areas favor it. *Enterobacter*, *Klebsiella*, *Escherichia coli*, and *Proteus* species are the predominant gram-negative organisms found on the skin. *Acinetobacter* is the major, gram-negative rod species on the skin. It may constitute about 25% of the total skin flora.

Bacterial Interference and Competition

Due to the massive numbers and variety of microbial species present on the skin surface, there is an intense competition for host resources and attachment sites. Bacteria are adept at impairing or killing other microbes to ensure their own species survival. The fitter genes are thus naturally selected and passed on to the next generation.

Bacterial interference refers to the phenomenon of antagonism that occurs between bacterial species during the process of surface colonization and ongoing fight for nutrients. Over time, bacteria have developed special mechanisms to interfere with the capability of their antagonistic bacteria to colonize and infect the host. This phenomenon has been extensively studied through prevention of colonization of nasal cavity by pathogens using *Corynebacterium* species, a common bacterium of the normal nasal flora. The artificially implanted strain of *Corynebacterium* species into the nares of 17 volunteers, who were carriers of *S. aureus*, showed that the *Corynebacterium* strain succeeded in eradicating the pathogen in 71% of the volunteers though a nonbacteriocin-like mechanism. Further evaluation showed the capacity of viridans streptococci to hinder colonization of the oral cavity of newborns by methicillin-resistant *S. aureus* (MRSA). Furthermore, *Lactobacillus* species is the predominant microorganism of the urogenital flora of healthy premenopausal women. Restoration of the normal flora by the use of locally or orally administered probiotics, based on the strains of *Lactobacillus* species, could protect against recurrence of urinary tract infection (UTI) and bacterial vaginosis. Thus, it is hypothesized that using interfering bacteria for preventive and/or therapeutic purposes is a valid approach. The preservation of existing microflora by avoiding smoking and broad-spectrum long-term antibiotic regimens thus becomes an effective modality for preventing infections.

Fungal Flora

Fungi are also common inhabitants of the skin surface, with yeasts being the predominant species.

Malassezia (Formerly known as Pityrosporum)

Malassezia (formerly known as *Pityrosporum*) is genus of fungi, naturally found on the skin surfaces of humans. They may cause occasional opportunistic infections. *Malassezia furfur* ubiquitously colonizes adults and even infants by the age of 3–6 months. There is seemingly no predilection for any particular age or sex. *Malassezia* (*Pityrosporum*) species, being lipophilic yeasts, are more prevalent in seborrheic areas. *Pityrosporum ovale* and *Pityrosporum orbiculare* are probably identical organisms that are prominent in sebaceous areas.

Candida

Candida species is another commensal present mostly in the oral mucous membranes (up to 40% of individuals). From this primary abode, it colonizes the vulvovaginal area. It has been estimated that 20% of asymptomatic healthy women of the childbearing group carry the infection, though it can vary between 10 and 50%. When a suitable opportunity presents, these vaginal species can become pathogenic and present with vulvovaginal candidiasis. When present on the skin, *Candida albicans* is the most common species found. Psoriatic, diabetic, atopic, and immunocompromised patients have a higher colonization of *Candida* in their skin and mucosa.

Viral Flora

A recent analysis of the human skin virome in healthy individuals and cancer patients has confirmed a flora dominated by human papilloma virus (HPV), human polyomaviruses (HPyV), and circoviruses.

Human papilloma virus was initially thought to be only present in skin cancer patients, but subsequently it was found that healthy skin is also a habitat for a broad spectrum of HPV strains. A diverse community of HPV types has been identified on healthy skin while identifying HPVs that were previously unknown.

The other major group of commensal human skin viruses is the HPyVs. Similar to HPV, HPyVs were originally studied in the context of cancer and were subsequently found on healthy human skin. The most common to human skin are HPyV6, HPyV7, and Merkel cell polyomavirus (MCPyV).

The other component of the human virome is the bacteriophage, about which little is known in the skin. Analysis of skin swabs from five healthy patients and one patient with a previous Merkel cell carcinoma lesion indicate that two families dominate cutaneous bacteriophage communities, the *Microviridae* and *Siphoviridae*. In the skin, bacteriophage communities have been suggested as mediators of resistance gene transfer between bacteria.

Parasites

Demodex is the genus of parasitic mites residing in or near hair follicles of mammals. These are among the smallest of arthropods, with two species typically found on humans. *Demodex* infestation is common in healthy adults (23-100%). *Demodex folliculorum* and *Demodex brevis* are typically found on the face (cheeks, nose, chin, forehead and temples), scalp, neck, and ears. These are the most common ectoparasite on the skin surface. They can be seen in 10% of skin biopsies. Although

D. folliculorum is the more common of the two mites, *D. brevis* has a wider distribution on the body. Prevalence of both species increases with age, with men being more heavily colonized than women (23% vs. 13%) and harboring more *D. brevis* than women (23% vs. 9%). Sebum appears to be essential for the survival of *Demodex*; hence, they are infrequent in infants and children. Penetration of *Demodex* into the dermis or more commonly an increase in the number of mites in the pilosebaceous unit (>5/cm^2) is thought to cause infestation, which triggers inflammation. Many facial conditions including rosacea, facial pruritus (with or without erythema), perioral dermatitis, Grover's disease, eosinophilic folliculitis, blepharitis, papulovesicular facial eruptions, papulopustular scalp eruptions, seborrheic dermatitis, etc., have higher colonization with *Demodex*. However, it remains unknown if *Demodex* is the causative factor or if *Demodex* mite density increases due to inflammation of affected follicles. Adding to the confusion is the fact that the clinical presentation of *Demodex* infestation is similar to that of rosacea and seborrheic dermatitis (SD) with facial flushing/blushing, erythema, telangiectasia, scaling and facial skin roughness on palpation, and centrofacial inflammatory lesions. There has been a suggestion that *Demodex* dermatitis may in fact be distinct from rosacea and SD. *Demodex* is not easily detected in histological preparations; therefore, the skin surface biopsy (SSB) technique with cyanoacrylic adhesion is a commonly used method to measure its density on the skin.

MEASUREMENT OF SKIN FLORA

Historically, characterizing the cutaneous microbes involved culturing skin swabs or biopsy specimens. However, less than 1% of bacterial species can be cultivated under standard laboratory conditions. Many of these that do grow are outcompeted by faster-growing organisms. Consequently, the more easily cultivated bacteria or fungi, such as *Staphylococcus* or *Malassezia* species, were overrepresented in early microbial surveys. Recent advances in deoxyribonucleic acid (DNA) amplification and sequencing technology have been able to bypass the need for culture, allowing a more complete and unbiased view of the skin microbiota and its genetic content.

Analysis of the bacterial microbiome is most often done by amplifying the prokaryotic small subunit ribosomal RNA (*16S rRNA*) gene by polymerase chain reaction (PCR), directly from the skin samples. The *16S rRNA* gene exists in all bacteria and archaea but not in eukaryotes.

Sequences that are more than 97% identical can often be classified within one species. In 2007, the National Institute of Health launched the Human Microbiome Project to survey the microbial content in healthy adults. This was to develop a reference catalog of the human microbial genome sequences. This involved the data from a population of 242 healthy adults, who were sampled at 15 or 18 body sites, up to three times. This generated 5,177 microbial taxonomic profiles from *16S rRNA* genes. Over 3.5 terabases of metagenomic sequence were published. The findings confirmed those of the previous smaller-scale studies, by suggesting that the skin microbiota is diverse, but dominated by a small group of genera, in particular *Staphylococcus, Cutibacterium*, and *Corynebacterium* (Human Microbiome Project Consortium 2012).

CHAPTER 2

Normal Oral Flora

Just like skin, the oral cavity is home to a multitude of microbes including many bacterial species. More than 700 bacterial species, of which over 50% have not been cultivated, have been detected in the oral cavity. Some of these bacteria have been implicated in the pathogenesis of oral diseases like caries and periodontitis (among the most common bacterial infections in humans).

Similar to the cutaneous ecological niches, oral cavity also allows preferential colonization in its various parts with varied surfaces. This is often a result of specific adhesins expressed on the bacterial surface, binding in turn to complementary specific receptors on oral mucosa. Six phyla of bacteria have been detected in the oral cavity. These include the Firmicutes (species of *Streptococcus, Gemella, Eubacterium, Selenomonas, Veillonella*, and related ones), the Actinobacteria (species of *Actinomyces, Atopobium, Rothia*, and related ones), the Proteobacteria (e.g., species of *Neisseria, Eikenella, Campylobacter*, and related ones), the Bacteroidetes (e.g., species of *Porphyromonas, Prevotella, Capnocytophaga*, and related ones), and the Fusobacteria (e.g., species of *Fusobacterium* and *Leptotrichia*). In their study, the most predominant bacterial genera were *Streptococcus, Gemella, Abiotrophia, Granulicatella, Rothia, Neisseria,* and *Prevotella*.

The role of bacteria in periodontal disease is complex. The presence of a high proportion of so-called red complex bacteria, i.e., *Porphyromonas gingivalis, Tannerella forsythia*, and *Treponema denticola*, is associated with periodontal disease. Oral spirochetes are present in the oral cavity in various numbers and forms and have been strongly implicated as playing a role in the etiology of periodontal disease. The great bulk of the literature concerns *T. denticola* and is most frequently isolated from severely diseased sites in young adults. Other spirochete species include *Borrelia refringens* and *Treponema macrodentium*.

CHAPTER 3

Factors Affecting the Skin Flora

INTRODUCTION

Skin flora is very dynamic, both in its constitution and composition. A variety of factors are known to affect the skin flora. These can be classified as endogenous or exogenous factors.

ENDOGENOUS FACTORS

Body site: The face, neck, and hands, being the exposed areas, have a higher proportion of transient organisms and a higher bacterial density. The face, scalp, and neck are sebaceous areas with a higher lipid content, and hence harbor *Cutibacterium* and *Malassezia* species. Intertriginous areas harbor almost all organisms; however, *Corynebacterium* and gram-negative rods are particularly common.

Effect of disease: The normal skin flora varies with comorbidities and diseases. For example, diabetics have a higher skin colonization with *Candida* and nasal colonization with *Staphylococcus aureus*, owing to increased skin glucose levels and immunosuppressive state.

Age: The skin flora changes as age progresses. Young children carry micrococci, coryneform bacteria, and gram-negative organisms more frequently, whereas *Pityrosporum* and *Cutibacterium* population increases with the onset of puberty.

Sex: Men are known to harbor more organisms. This could be due to their higher sebum secretion rates, higher sweat production, and more occlusive clothing in general.

EXOGENOUS FACTORS (ENVIRONMENTAL)

Temperature: Higher temperatures and higher humidity levels provide the requisite environment for bacteria as well as fungi to multiply. This is possibly the reason for more skin infections in the tropical climate. Keeping the skin surface cool and dry is known to effectively prevent skin infections.

Hospitalization: The skin of hospitalized patients has been shown to harbor nosocomial flora like *Corynebacterium, Proteus, Pseudomonas, Candida albicans* and *S. aureus*. This is attributable to an increased exposure to often resistant bacteria, coupled with the patient's ill-health. Hospital workers are also known to be prone to acquire nosocomial organisms and staphylococcal carriage.

Occupation: Occupations involving exposure to higher temperatures and wearing of occlusive clothing favor increased growth of organisms, particularly those that grow in a moist environment.

Soaps and disinfectants: Overzealous washing of face or hands is a commonly encountered habit. This disturbs the skin pH and often strips the acid mantle leading to growth of organisms like *Cutibacterium*. Thus, it is a sound advice to use mildly acidic face washes in acne. Deliberate reduction of skin surface bacteria with agents like chlorhexidine is a commonly practiced approach to reduce the incidence of postoperative infections. It has been shown to decrease postoperative infections caused by *S. aureus* from 8 to 2%.

Effect of cosmetics: Some cosmetic formulations are formulated to contain antimicrobial agents. A prolonged use of such products may promote resistance among the resident microflora. The use of antiseptic and medicated soaps, apart from other cosmetics like deodorants and body sprays, protects the skin by controlling the population of microorganisms. A higher number of microbes have been documented on the skin surface of people using coconut oil [90.4×10^2 colony-forming units (CFUs)/5 cm^2 skin area]. The microbial count of persons using and not using cosmetics has been found to be 34.4×10^2 and 45.6×10^2 CFU/5 cm^2 area of skin surface, respectively. It has been reported that deodorants have a bacteriostatic effect on skin microflora. A positive correlation has been observed between body odor and prevalence of skin flora and with the use and nonuse of deodorants. A combination of alcohol with any antimicrobial lotion enhances its antimicrobial activity as a synergistic effect. Spray deodorants have a greater antimicrobial effect than the gel and stick types. This could be attributed to the alcohol base used in spray-type deodorants. Alcohol and propellants like butane or propane provide better results, probably due to the better and exaggerated exposure of microbes to the antimicrobial agents and also due to their better penetration into fat/sebaceous glands, skin, ducts, dead cells and follicles.

Effects of medications: Drugs alter the normal skin flora to a great extent. The alteration is further enhanced by dermatological therapeutics involving the use of immunosuppressants for long periods. This leads to a suppression of the normal skin flora, encouraging the growth of pathogenic strains. Drugs also alter the nasal flora. A reduction in coryneform counts with a corresponding increase in coagulase-negative micrococci and gram-negative organisms is known to occur. Women on estrogens have also been documented to have a higher incidence of vaginal candidiasis. Studies with isotretinoin intake have shown a decreased colonization with *Propionibacterium acnes*. The number of gram-negative rods decreases significantly and *S. aureus* colonization of the anterior nares and the skin is increased. Nasal decolonization with topical antibiotics is thus a useful adjunct to therapy with oral retinoids. Even topical therapy with antibiotics in acne leads to alteration of the skin flora and consequent drug resistance. Long-term antibiotics are often given in acne. It is now known that in the gut, these antibiotics cause not only a transient loss in bacterial diversity but also a long-term loss of normal gut flora beyond the direct antibiotic targets. This may cause unknown changes in the gut flora beyond the target organisms and in turn modify disease recurrence.

CHAPTER 4

Skin Flora in Disease

INTRODUCTION

Apart from physiological variations, disease states are also known to alter skin flora. This may have a special implication with respect to fungal infections. Various disease states are associated with alterations in the resident flora, which could be both a cause and a result of the disease process. Such alterations are summarized in the following text **(Fig. 1)**.

SKIN FLORA IN ATOPIC DERMATITIS

Atopic dermatitis is known to flare with a change in the microbial environment of the skin. Currently, the data on probiotics in the management of skin disease remains controversial. However, a recent meta-analysis of six randomized controlled trials shows that the use of probiotics decreased SCORAD (Scoring Atopic Dermatitis) significantly in adult patients with atopic dermatitis, improving their quality of life. Topical steroids, however, do not alter the flora to any significant extent and might even help in reducing the pathogenic flora in eczematous conditions such as atopic dermatitis. Effective treatments for atopic dermatitis, such as antibiotics and steroids, are thought to work by decreasing the bacterial load and inhibiting a dysfunctional, exuberant immune response to skin flora. Colonization by *Staphylococcus aureus* is one of the various hypotheses suggested in the pathogenesis of atopic dermatitis. A subset of patients with atopic dermatitis of the head and neck has been found to have *Malassezia* flora fueling their disease.

CHAPTER 4: Skin Flora in Disease

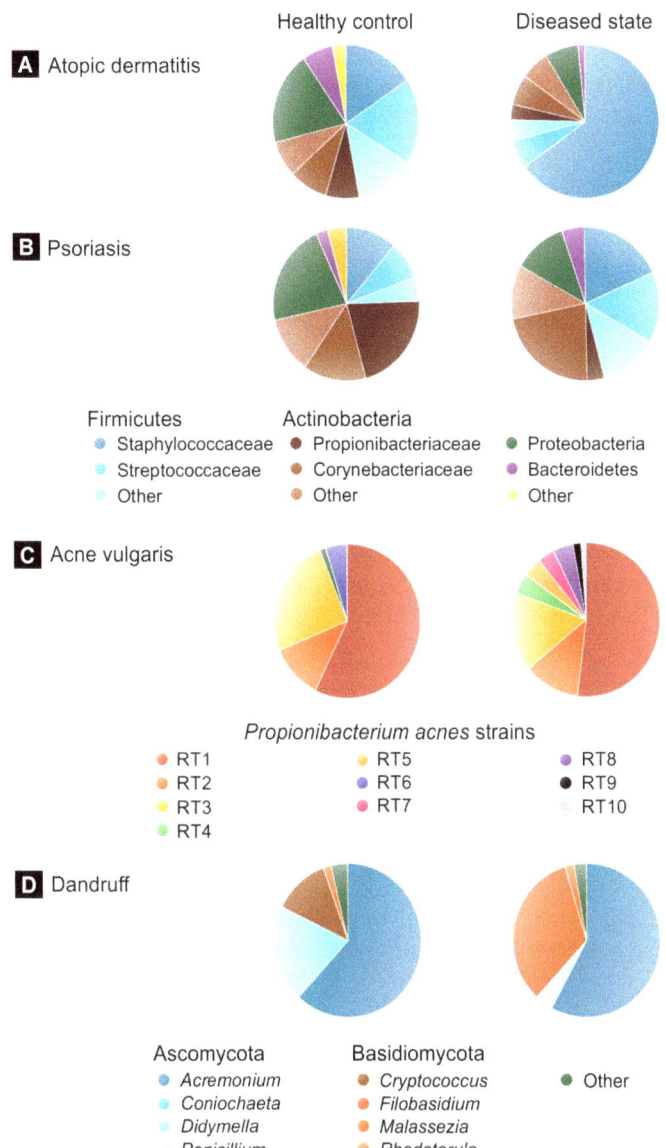

Figs. 1A to D: Changes in skin microbiota associated with disease states. (A) Relative abundance of bacteria (16S rRNA) in 12 children with atopic dermatitis flares as compared with 11 healthy controls. (B) Relative abundance of bacteria (16S rRNA) in six patients with psoriasis, in the lesional area as compared with unaffected skin as a control. (C) Relative abundance of *Propionibacterium acnes* strains in 49 acne patients and 52 healthy individuals. (D) Relative abundance of fungi (26S rRNA) in three healthy scalps and four dandruff-afflicted scalps.

SKIN FLORA IN ACNE

Follicular flora in acne predominantly consists of *Cutibacterium acnes*. Topical and systemic antibacterial drugs have long been used to treat acne, with the efficacy commonly attributed to decreased *C. acnes* colonization and/or activity.

SKIN FLORA IN PSORIASIS

Multiple clinical observations support a role for imbalance of the skin microbiota in the pathogenesis of psoriasis. This includes the clinical efficacy of topical corticosteroids in the treatment of psoriasis. Early culture-based studies examining microorganisms associated with psoriasis identified *Malassezia*, group A and B β-hemolytic streptococci, *S. aureus,* and *Enterococcus faecalis*. Analyses of the bacterial microbiota by *16S rRNA* gene-based approaches in cross-sectional studies suggest an underrepresentation of *Cutibacterium* and an increased representation of the phylum Firmicutes in the psoriatic plaques, as compared with healthy controls or uninvolved limb skin.

SKIN FLORA IN SEBORRHEIC DERMATITIS

It has been found that dandruff-afflicted skin harbors relative abundances of *Malassezia* species. Increased numbers of *Penicillium* and *Filobasidium floriforme* have also been documented that correlates with an increased severity of dandruff. Furthermore, it has been suggested that because *Malassezia* is found in the commensal fungal microbiota, it is not likely to be causing the disease on its own. There may be other interactive mechanisms involved in etiopathogenesis.

ROLE OF SKIN FLORA IN DEVELOPING IMMUNITY

Evidence suggests that both skin and gut microbiota play a crucial role in educating and assisting the immune system. A recent study has shown that germ-free mice, without commensal skin microbes, have abnormal cytokine production and cutaneous T-cell populations. Healthy skin barrier consists of both immune surveillance and epidermal keratinocytes, which produce antimicrobial peptides that contribute not only to the innate immunity but also to the adaptive immunity. Expression of these antimicrobial peptides are upregulated by the presence of

Cutibacterium species and other gram-positive bacteria. In addition to the antimicrobial peptides, sebocytes also produce antimicrobial free-fatty acids by hydrolyzing sebum triglycerides. This triglyceride hydrolysis is also performed by commensal bacterial flora such as *Propionibacterium acnes* and *Staphylococcus epidermidis*. The effect of skin microbiota on the innate and adaptive immune system is an area of active investigation because many diseases such as dermatomyositis, and lupus, to name a few, manifest on the skin, even if they are also systemic.

ROLE OF SKIN FLORA IN CANCER IMMUNOLOGY

Cancers are known to occur with loss of immune surveillance. Because the skin microbiome is important for developing a well-functioning immune system and for modulating inflammation, it may also have a protective role against some cancers. Studies have shown that workers such as farmers and waste-incinerator workers, who were exposed heavily to the environmental microbiota, have lower cancer rates.

SECTION 2

Dermatophytosis

Chapter 5: Epidemiology and Etiology of Dermatophytosis in India
Chapter 6: Pathogenesis of Dermatophytosis
Chapter 7: Dermatophytosis of Skin
Chapter 8: Recalcitrant Dermatophytosis
Chapter 9: Tinea Capitis
Chapter 10: Onychomycosis

CHAPTER 5

Epidemiology and Etiology of Dermatophytosis in India

INTRODUCTION

Superficial dermatophytosis has become the most commonly encountered infection in the clinical practice. What was once considered as benign and easy-to-treat infection, mainly seen during summer and rainy season, has now become a perennial and difficult-to-treat disease. There has been a sudden increase in its incidence all over the country in the last one decade. This increase has been at an alarming rate and has gained the proportion of an epidemic-like situation. The current scenario has become worse by the increase in the incidence of chronic, relapsing, and recurrent dermatophytosis.

EPIDEMIOLOGY

There is paucity of community-based surveys and most numbers come from hospital-based studies. A prevalence of 27.6% to 32% has been reported for dermatophytosis in studies from South India with hot and humid weather that is conducive to the growth of fungus. On the contrary, a high prevalence of 61.5% has been recorded from North India that has winter season lasting for 5–6 months. In majority of tertiary care hospitals, approximately 30–50% of dermatology outpatients present with dermatophytosis.

Age and Gender

Conventionally, adult men are more frequently affected than women simply because of significantly high incidence of *tinea cruris*, *tinea pedis*, and *tinea unguium* in men. Outdoor working with hot, humid, and sweaty conditions put men and women at risk of dermatophytosis. However, in the present epidemic, there is a rising incidence of dermatophytosis across all age groups including infants, young children and old age. It is common to see close family members, especially the close contacts like spouse and young children to have concomitant infection. It will not be an exaggeration to state that dermatophytosis is considered "new scabies." Therefore, a careful enquiry into the family history has become the usual norm in order to treat all the affected family members simultaneously in order to prevent chronicity and recurrences.

Topical Steroid Abuse

Usual treatment modalities for dermatophytosis or tinea include either topical or systemic antifungal drugs or a combination of both. In last one decade, innumerable fixed-drug combination containing potent topical steroid (clobetasol propionate) with antifungal, antibiotic, antiprotozoal have become available over the counter and are being used for dermatophytosis indiscriminately and erratically over months and years, often suggested by the pharmacists and friends. This has led to the development of steroid-modified tinea (tinea incognito) which is extensive and difficult to diagnose due to atypical morphology. This form is more likely to become chronic, resistant, and relapsing in nature and adversely affects the quality of life.

ETIOLOGY OF SUPERFICIAL DERMATOPHYTOSIS

In the present epidemic of superficial dermatophytosis, the etiological fungus has undergone a tremendous epidemiological shift from *Trichophyton rubrum (T. rubrum)* most prevalent until 2011 to *T. mentagrophytes* (also referred to as *T. mentagrophytes/T. interdigitale* complex) which has now emerged as the predominant organism. *T. mentagrophytes* exhibits a rapid growth in primary culture within 5–7 days; this might explain the extensive involvement, inflammatory lesions, and fomite transmission frequently seen now. It is an anthropophilic species, spreading from human to human. The molecular identification by polymerase chain reaction (PCR)-based sequencing of the rDNA has identified this fungus to be *T. mentagrophytes* ITS genotype VIII, also being referred as *T. indotineae*.

CHAPTER 6

Pathogenesis of Dermatophytosis

INTRODUCTION

Dermatophytes are a group of related fungi capable of breaking down and digesting the keratin in skin, hair, and nails. These are mostly environmental pathogens, but based on their preferred habitat or ecological niche, they can be classified as geophilic, anthropophilic, and zoophilic dermatophytes **(Table 1)**.

The initial source of infection are the arthroconidia or spores of the infective species, deposited on the surface of the host (skin, hair or nails). The dermatophyte, thus, colonizes the stratum corneum and starts using keratin as the source of its nutrition.

Under normal circumstances, the dermatophyte hyphae or mycelium is incapable of penetrating the viable layers of skin. This implies that their in-vivo activity is restricted to specific zones. These include the newly differentiated keratin of skin; the nail plate structure (thick keratin), and the area above the Adamson's fringe within the hair shaft.

Under favorable circumstances, the inoculated arthroconidia undergo the following well-characterized phases of growth. These are responsible for the clinical manifestations of the fungal infection of skin and its appendages.

- *Adherence:* The arthroconidia adhere to individual keratinocytes through yet unknown mediators. In-vitro models have revealed the presence of fibril-like structures on the arthroconidia that help them in attaching to the keratinocyte surface. A firm adherence is followed by the germination of the arthroconidia into hyphal element.

TABLE 1: Medically significant dermatophyte species with their favored ecological niche.

Dermatophyte species	Habitat	Mode of transmission	Immune response	Worldwide cases
Geophilic species (originating in soil) • *Microsporum gypseum* • *Microsporum praecox*	Soil	Contact with soil	Inflammatory	Sporadic
Anthropophilic species (largely restricted to humans) • *Epidermophyton floccosum* • *Microsporum audouinii var. rivalieri* • *Microsporum audouinii var. langeronii* • *Microsporum ferrugineum* • *Trichophyton concentricum* • *Trichophyton gourville* • *Trichophyton mentagrophytes var. interdigitale* • *Trichophyton megnini* • *Trichophyton rubrum* • *Trichophyton schoenleinii* • *Trichophyton soudanense* • *Trichophyton tonsurans* • *Trichophyton violaceum* • *Trichophyton yaounde*	Humans	Direct contact or fomites	Varies, noninflammatory to inflammatory	Epidemic

Continued

CHAPTER 6: Pathogenesis of Dermatophytosis

Continued

Dermatophyte species	Habitat	Mode of transmission	Immune response	Worldwide cases
Zoophilic (commonly infecting animals) • *Microsporum canis* var. *canis* • *Microsporum canis* var. *distortum* • *Microsporum equinum* • *Microsporum gallinae* • *Microsporum incanum* • *Microsporum versicolor* • *Trichophyton equinum* • *Trichophyton mentagrophytes* var. *mentagrophytes,* var. *erinacei,* var. *quinckeanum* • *Trichophyton simii* • *Trichophyton verrucosum*	Animals (cats, dogs)	Direct contact with animal or indirectly through infected hair in the clothing	Inflammatory (spontaneous cure may occur)	Sporadic

- *Penetration:* The dermatophyte hyphae produce an arsenal of proteases, which are capable of breaking down keratin, which is their main source of nutrition. It is postulated that mechanical factors may also play a role in this invasion. The site preference exhibited by certain dermatophyte species (e.g., *Epidermophyton floccosum* rarely infecting the hair follicle and occasionally infecting the nail) may be explained on the basis of this selective step.
- *Host response*: Fungal penetration and growth invokes the host immune response. Both innate as well as acquired immunity are involved. Antimicrobial peptides such as cathelicidins and human beta-defensins are proposed to be the main factors involved in the innate response to fungal invasion. They have antifungal activity. Additionally, certain serum factors such as transferrins also have an inhibitory effect on fungal growth. The fungi also have chemotactic properties and can activate the alternate pathway of the complement system.

The cell-mediated immune response against fungi is the one that is primarily protective. It is a delayed type of hypersensitivity response. Dermatophyte antigens are taken up by the Langerhans cell present in the epidermis. These are then carried to the local lymph nodes, where they are presented to CD4+ T-lymphocytes. The exposed and sensitized T-lymphocytes proliferate in turn, migrate back to the dermis to produce an inflammatory response. Patients with widespread dermatophyte infection may also have detectable levels of antibodies to the dermatophyte antigen. However, this humoral immunity does not appear to be protective against the spread of the infection.

This simple model of pathogenesis of dermatophyte infection is in turn affected by many other factors. These include the host's age, sex, race, rate of sebum production (sebum has inhibitory action on dermatophyte proliferation), break in the skin barrier, immune status, glucocorticoid usage, etc. All these may affect the clinical response of the host and the clinical pattern of presentation. An association between atopy (characterized by increased IgE levels) and chronic dermatophytic infection has also been reported.

IMMUNOPATHOGENESIS OF CHRONIC DERMATOPHYTOSIS

In certain cases, the fungi are able to effectively evade the host immune response, enabling them to thrive and produce a chronic infection. They employ various protective mechanisms to produce this scenario including a masking of the cell wall-associated carbohydrates, or an effective shielding of the surface recognition molecules, which otherwise play a stimulatory role. Toll-like receptor recognition along with a downregulation of the complement cascade. A higher expression of T helper 17 (Th17) and regulatory T (Treg) cell markers has been documented on the CD4+ cells of patients with chronic dermatophytosis in comparison to classical tinea. This altered Th17/Treg ratio in patients with chronic infection is likely to be responsible for a poor treatment response as well, as it prevents effective fungal clearance.

CHAPTER 7

Dermatophytosis of Skin

INTRODUCTION

Dermatophytoses are superficial fungal infections caused by dermatophytes. These are a group of molds which are predominantly environmental pathogens belonging mostly to various asexual genera. Some of the species may be zoophilic or anthropophilic as well. This chapter discusses the various skin manifestations of dermatophytosis.

Traditionally, the dermatophytoses are classified based on the body site involved. This includes tinea corporis, tinea barbae, tinea faciei, tinea capitis, tinea pedis, tinea manuum, tinea cruris, and tinea unguium. Owing to the unique characteristics afforded by the different sites involved, the clinical manifestations vary accordingly.

TINEA CORPORIS

It is the dermatophytic infection of the glabrous skin (free from hair) except for the skin of palms, soles, and groins. It is usually seen in individuals residing in areas with hot and humid climates. Although, it can occur in all age groups, it is more common in adults.

Etiopathogenesis

Although all dermatophyte species are reported to cause tinea corporis; the most common species isolated are *Trichophyton rubrum*, *T. mentagrophytes*, *Microsporum canis*, and *M. tonsurans*.

Incubation Period

Post inoculation, the reported incubation period is 1–3 weeks.

Clinical Features

The clinical presentations may vary depending on the causative species as well as host immunity. Itching is mostly present and may be quite severe. In less inflammatory cases, there are characteristic annular plaques with raised erythematous borders **(Fig. 1)**. The central clearing seen is due to the inflammatory response against the pathogenic fungi causing the fungi to migrate centrifugally within the horny layer of the epidermis. However, this characteristic central clearing may not always be present. The presence of scales at the erythematous borders can generally be appreciated in treatment-naïve cases. In severe inflammatory cases, there may be vesicles and/or pustules at the margin, instead of scales. Rarely, bulla formation can also occur, especially with *T. rubrum*.

Apart from this prototype presentation of tinea corporis, other special types have also been described in the following text.

- Tinea faciei (dermatophytic infection of the skin of the face) is most commonly caused by *T. rubrum* and *T. mentagrophytes*. In these cases, apart from itching, the patient may complain of significant burning sensation after exposure to the sun. These lesions are frequently modified by application of topical corticosteroids **(Fig. 2)**.

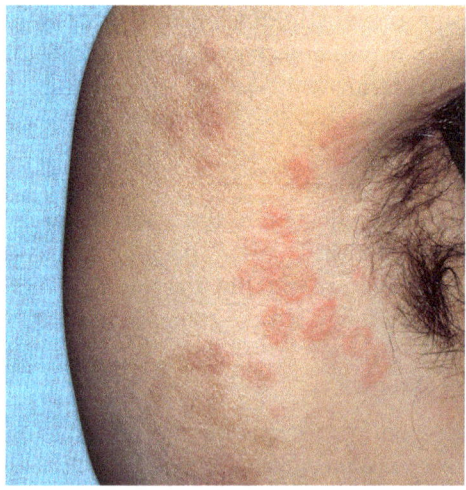

Fig. 1: Annular lesions of tinea corporis.

CHAPTER 7: Dermatophytosis of Skin

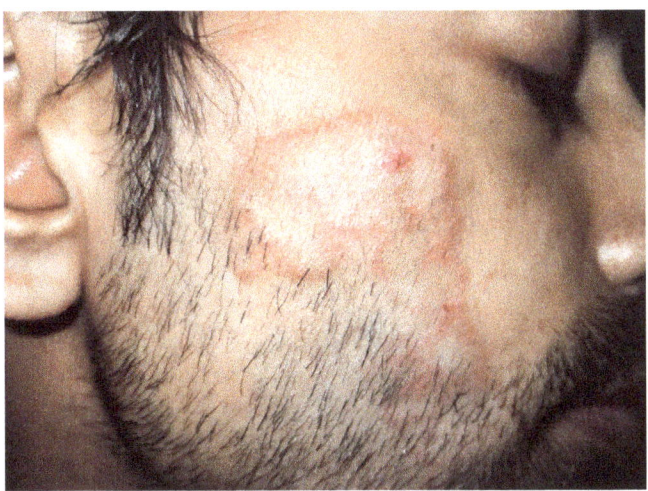

Fig. 2: Tinea faciei in a young male.

- Tinea imbricata is a special subtype, caused by the species *T. concentricum* (anthropophilic). This form is especially reported from South Asia, Mexico, and Brazil. It presents as multiple, concentric, and polycyclic erythematous lesions with scales at the border. This type of tinea corporis is usually chronic and may involve the whole body. This dramatic clinical picture is associated with negative delayed type hypersensitivity to *T. concentricum* antigen.
- Tinea indecisiva (commonly caused by *T. mentagrophytes* and *T. tonsurans*) clinically manifest as erythematous annular plaques with multiple concentric rings within the plaque. This morphology resembles tinea imbricata caused by *T. concentricum* **(Fig. 3)**. Long-term cyclical therapy with topical antifungals and/or corticosteroids may produce this manifestation. This occurs due to similar underlying mechanisms of immunosuppression with the use of topical corticosteroids and reinfection due to an early discontinuation of topical antifungals.
- Majocchi granuloma is a type of deep fungal folliculitis, most commonly seen in women who regularly shave their hair. It presents as perifollicular pustules and nodules with surrounding erythema **(Fig. 4)**. It is most commonly caused by *T. rubrum*.

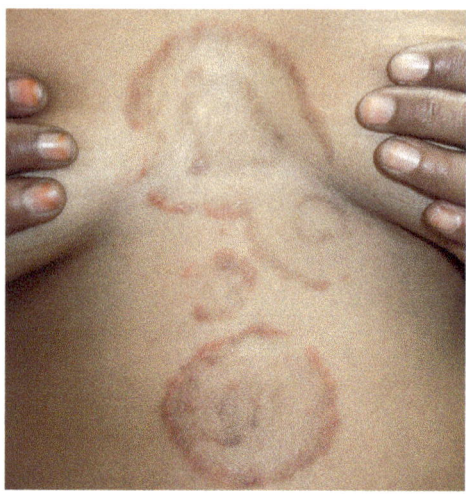

Fig. 3: Concentric rings in a case of tinea indecisiva, extensive involvement over the trunk can be seen.

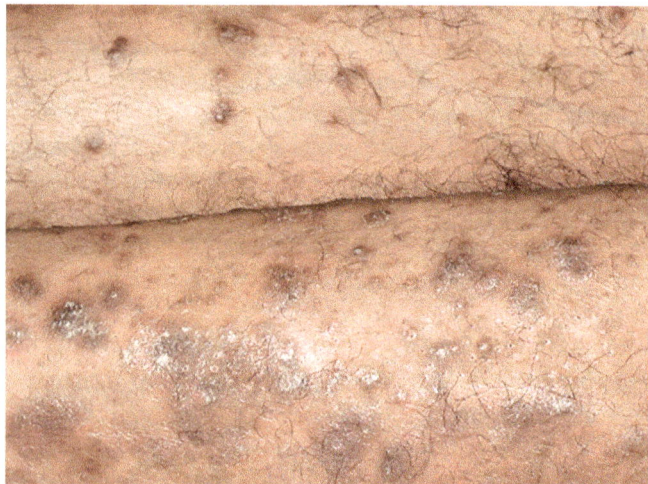

Fig. 4: Deep-seated inflammation on the legs in a case with extensive tinea corporis.

- Tinea incognito (tinea modified by topical or systemic corticosteroids) is generally a result of suppression of inflammation. It can be difficult to recognize due to an absence of the characteristic raised margins and scales **(Fig. 5)**.

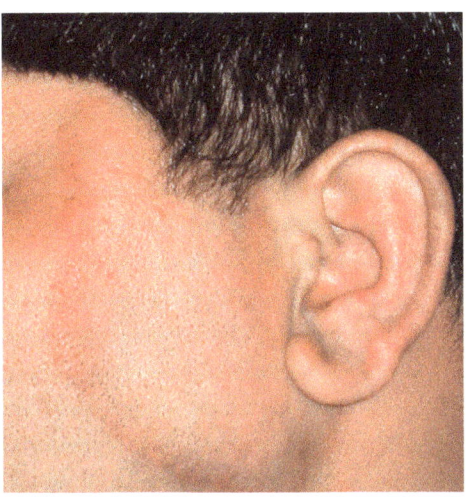

Fig. 5: Steroid-modified tinea or tinea incognito. Note the minimal to absent scaling.

Other rare forms described in literature are agminate folliculitis (plaque studded with pustules at the periphery) and subcutaneous abscesses.

Differential Diagnosis

The differential diagnoses are summarized in **Box 1**.

BOX 1	Differential diagnosis of tinea corporis.
• Seborrheic dermatitis	• Pityriasis rosea
• Psoriasis	• Secondary syphilis
• Annular erythema	• Subacute lupus erythematosus
• Pityriasis versicolor	

TINEA CRURIS OR DHOBI ITCH

This is an infection of the groin, perianal, and perineal areas caused by dermatophytes. It is more commonly seen in young males and is commoner in hot climates. The condition is more common in summer months and is associated with increased sweating and heavy manual work.

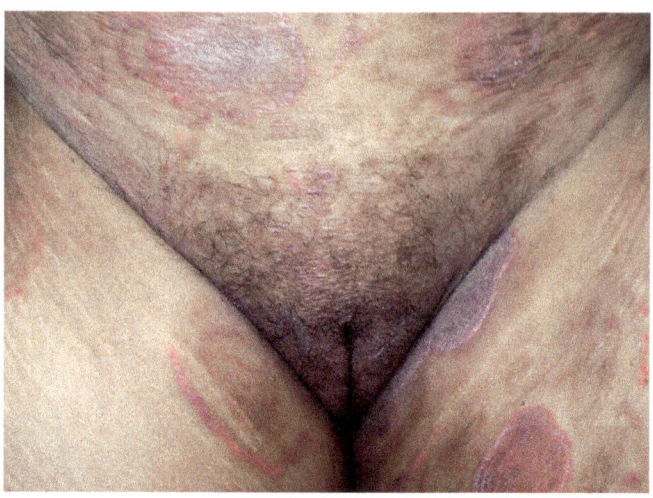

Fig. 6: Tinea cruris with involvement of groins. Extensive areas of involvement can be seen.

Etiopathogenesis

Although *T. rubrum* is most commonly implicated, *T. mentagrophytes* var. interdigitale and *Epidermophyton floccosum* may also be involved in some cases. The infection is a result of the moist conditions in the folds along with chronic friction.

Clinical Features

Although, the morphology is similar to tinea corporis, maceration is a more prominent feature. Superadded bacterial infection may also develop. The lesions are highly pruritic **(Fig. 6)**. Infection with *T. rubrum* may spread from groins to thighs, lower abdomen, back and buttocks. It has been seen that tinea cruris caused by *E. floccosum* infection is generally associated with concomitant foot involvement; while *T. mentagrophytes var. interdigitale* infection presents with more inflammation and a vesico-pustular margin.

Differential Diagnosis

The differential diagnoses are summarized in **Box 2**. Candidal intertrigo may be a common confusion; however, the clinical clues towards it being tinea cruris include the presence of well-defined borders, less maceration, more scales and absence of satellite pustules. Some cases

BOX 2	Differential diagnosis of tinea cruris.
• Candidal intertrigo • Erythrasma • Pityriasis versicolor	• Flexural psoriasis • Seborrheic dermatitis

of erythrasma and pityriasis versicolor may also be confused with tinea cruris, though the two conditions do not show central clearing and are not as symptomatic or itchy. Flexural psoriasis and seborrheic dermatitis may also mimic tinea cruris. Dermoscopy can help differentiate at times.

TINEA BARBAE

Tinea infection of the beard and moustache area is known as tinea barbae. It is more commonly seen in adult males. It is commoner in rural areas due to higher incidence of contact with animals, especially livestock. It can also be transmitted through barbers because of the use of shared razors.

Etiopathogenesis

Tinea barbae is most commonly caused by *T. mentagrophytes* and *T. verrucosum* (zoophilic species). Occasionally other species including *M. canis, T. violaceum,* and *T. schoenleinii* may also be responsible.

Clinical Presentation

Tinea barbae typically presents as multiple folliculocentric papules and pustules with surrounding erythema **(Fig. 7)**. There is associated exudation and crusting, quite resembling inflammatory tinea of the scalp. The hairs in the involved area are easily pluckable. Chronic cases may present with abscess and sinus formation, ultimately leading to scarring. Infection with anthropophilic species is often associated with less of inflammatory change. In such cases, circular, scaly plaques may be seen.

Differential Diagnosis

The differential diagnoses for tinea barbae are summarized in **Box 3**. The inflammatory variant of tinea barbae needs to be distinguished from sycosis barbae (deep folliculitis caused by *Staphylococcus aureus*).

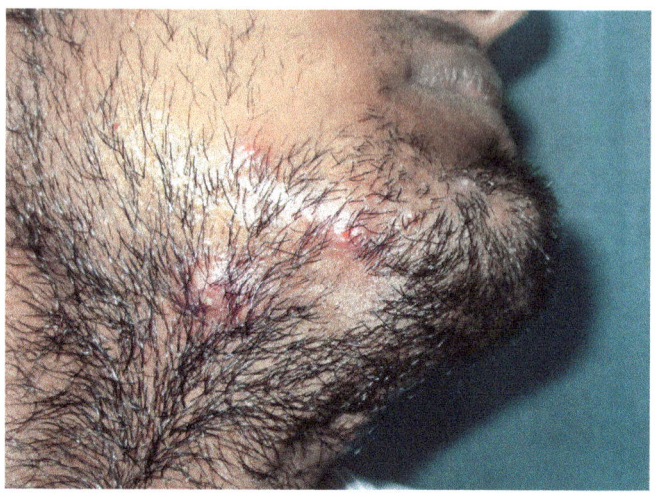

Fig. 7: Tinea barbae with marked inflammation. Deep-seated lesions with scarring can be appreciated in the beard area.

BOX 3	Differential diagnosis of tinea barbae.
• Sycosis barbae	• Rosacea
• Acne vulgaris	• Perioral dermatitis

Sycosis barbae is relatively more painful. Also, the hair in the center of the pustule is only occasionally loosened up. Acne vulgaris, papulopustular stage of rosacea, or cases of perioral dermatitis may mimic the less inflammatory variants of tinea barbae.

TINEA PEDIS OR ATHLETE'S FOOT

Tinea pedis refers to a superficial fungal infection of the foot and toes caused by dermatophytes. It is a condition which is often chronic, may be less symptomatic, and particularly common in patients engaging in wet work or wearing occlusive footwear.

Etiopathogenesis

The fungal species commonly isolated from cases with tinea pedis include *T. rubrum, T. mentagrophytes var. interdigitale,* and *E. floccosum.* There is

CHAPTER 7: Dermatophytosis of Skin

TABLE 1: Clinical variants of tinea pedis.

Clinical type	Implicated species	Clinical features
Chronic interdigital tinea pedis **(Fig. 8)**	• *Trichophyton rubrum* • *T. mentagrophytes var. interdigitale* • *Epidermophyton floccosum*	Erythema, maceration, and erosion of the toe cleft may extend to involve the undersurface of foot
Chronic hyperkeratotic type or Moccasin type of tinea pedis **(Fig. 9)**	*T. rubrum*	• Diffuse scaling of the sole extending to involve the medial and lateral surface of foot; erythema is variable, involvement is often bilateral • Involvement of one hand and two feet is known as "one-hand and two-feet syndrome" **(Fig. 11)**
Vesiculobullous type of tinea pedis	*T. mentagrophytes var. interdigitale*	• Multiple tense vesicles or vesicopustules on the sole and periplantar region rupture to leave behind a collarette of scale; bullae may also form • Spontaneous resolution can occur

a possibility of mixed infection as well, with two fungi being isolated from the same lesion.

Clinical Features

Tinea pedis can present as one of the three clinical variants or combined infections **(Table 1)**. The same are depicted in **Figures 8 and 9**.

TINEA MANUUM

Dermatophytes infection of the skin of the hands is known as tinea manuum. The condition, when presenting on the dorsum of the hand, may present similar to tinea corporis. The palmar infection is associated with diffuse scaling accentuated at the creases **(Fig. 10)**. Most of the cases are unilateral. Commonly, there is "one-hand, two-feet involvement" with dermatophytes **(Fig. 11)**.

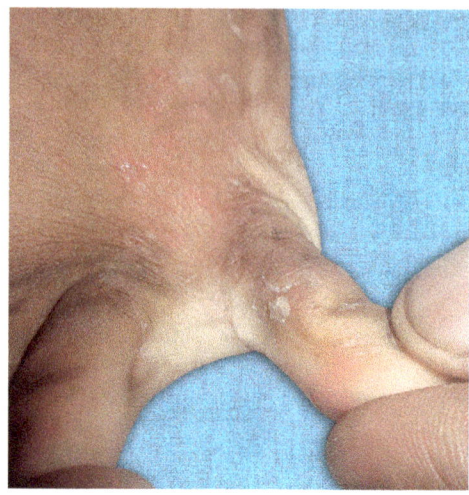

Fig. 8: Interdigital tinea pedis. The erythematous scaly plaque is involving the last interdigital cleft—an area of predilection.

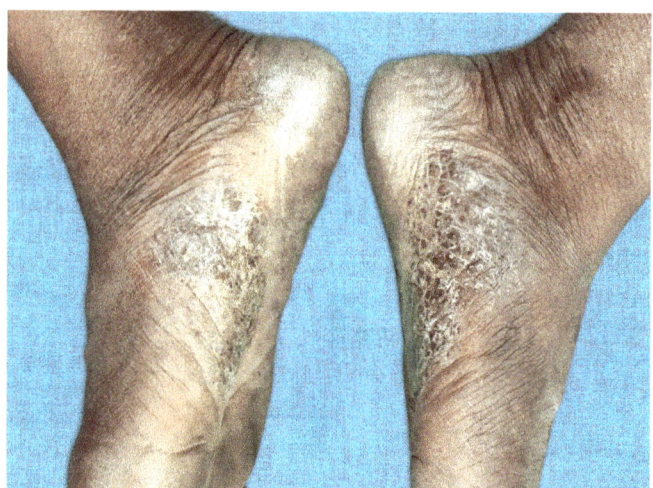

Fig. 9: Moccasin type, chronic hyperkeratotic tinea pedis. Note the extension of erythema and scaling from the plantar aspect along the lateral border of the foot.

CHAPTER 7: Dermatophytosis of Skin

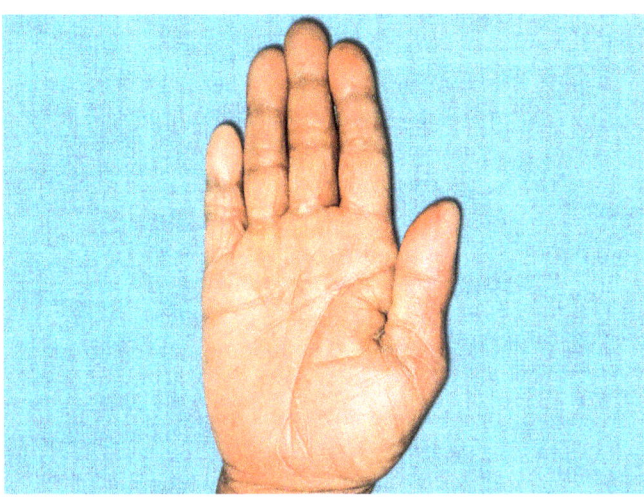

Fig. 10: Tinea manuum, chronic scaly hyperkeratosis involving the palmar as well as dorsal aspect of the hand.

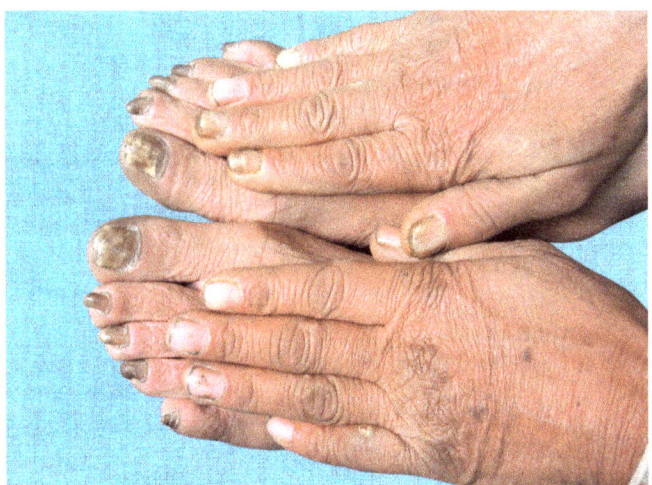

Fig. 11: One-hand and two-feet involvement in dermatophytosis.

DERMATOPHYTID REACTIONS

Dermatophytid refers to the cutaneous eruption occurring as a hypersensitivity response to a distant focus of dermatophyte infection. These skin eruptions are not infective by themselves, but are usually associated with a severe inflammatory dermatophytic infection occurring at a distant primary site. Most often, the primary infection is a kerion (inflammatory tinea capitis).

The clinical presentation of a dermatophytid reaction may vary from widespread follicular papules to pompholyx-like lesions **(Fig. 12)**. Some cases of erythema nodosum have also been reported with kerion as the primary.

The management of dermatophytids includes treatment of the primary focus of infection. This leads to a resolution of the id eruption. Topical corticosteroids and oral antihistaminics can be used to provide symptomatic relief to the patient.

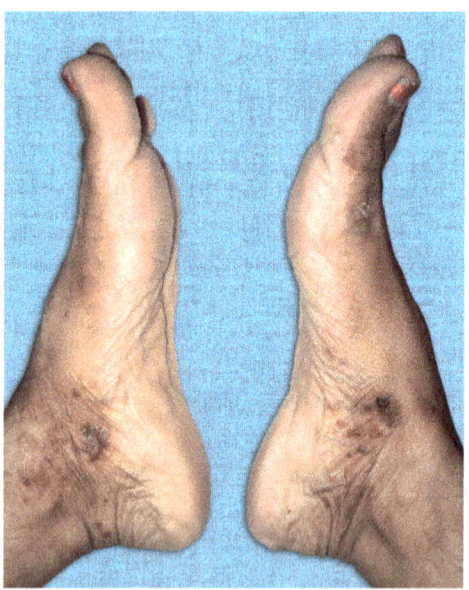

Fig. 12: Pompholyx-like inflammatory lesions acrally in a child with kerion.

TRICHOPHYTON RUBRUM SYNDROME

This syndrome refers to a chronic, widespread dermatophyte infection. It has been defined as a combination of multiple site involvement with *T. rubrum*. The following three criteria are required for a diagnosis:
1. Skin lesions at the following four sites:
   a. Feet, often involving soles
   b. Hands, often involving palms
   c. Nails
   d. At least one lesion in location other than these a, b, c sites, except for the groin
2. Positive microscopic analysis of potassium hydroxide preparations of skin scrapings in all four locations
3. Identification of *T. rubrum* by fungal culture at three of the four locations at least.

The syndrome has been associated with a *Trichophyton*-specific functional defect of phagocytic function, making the patient more prone to develop widespread dermatophyte infection, without other signs of immunodeficiency. It may represent a distinct clinical entity.

CHAPTER 8

Recalcitrant Dermatophytosis

INTRODUCTION

Recalcitrant dermatophytosis refers to the relapse, recurrence, reinfection, persistence, and possibly microbiological resistance of dermatophytosis. Over the past decade, cutaneous dermatophytoses have assumed epidemic proportions. We are witnessing much more severe and extensive fungal infections. Treatment-resistant tinea infections have been becoming extremely common. We are seeing atypical and extensive disease presentations. There has been an increase in chronic, relapsing, and recurrent cases.

In the context of this growing menace of superficial dermatophytosis, it is important to define few terms as per literature:
- *Chronic dermatophytosis* refers to a patient who has suffered from the disease for >6 months to 1 year duration, with or without recurrence, in spite of being treated.
- *Recurrent dermatophytosis* refers to the recurrence of the dermatophyte infection within 6 weeks of stopping the adequate antifungal treatment with at least two such episodes in last 6 months.
- *Recalcitrant dermatophytosis*: This unifying umbrella term encompasses both chronic and recurrent dermatophytosis clubbed together.

CHANGES IN THE PATTERN OF TINEA INFECTIONS

In today's scenario, the following changes are being increasingly observed pertaining to superficial dermatophytotic infections **(Box 1)**. These are also responsible for major challenges in their management and are detailed in the following text.

CHAPTER 8: Recalcitrant Dermatophytosis

> **BOX 1** **Changing patterns of superficial dermatophytosis.**
>
> - *Involvement of unusual locations*:
>   - Rising incidence of tinea faciei
>   - Tinea genitalis (males and females)
>   - Superficial dermatophytosis of scalp skin
>   - Tinea auricularis
>   - Tinea labialis
>   - Tinea ciliaris and tinea blepharitis
>   - Tinea of vellus hair
>   - Tinea involving immune compromised districts
> - *Changes in morphology*:
>   - Tinea pseudoimbricata
>   - Arcuate, dumbbell-shaped tinea corporis
>   - Large, bizarre-shaped or geographic patches of tinea corporis
>   - Double-edged tinea
>   - Ill-defined and unclear borders
>   - Eczematous tinea
>   - Tinea mimicking other dermatoses
> - *Changes in clinical behavior*:
>   - Unusually extensive diseases with or without comorbidity
>   - Multifocal disease at presentation
>   - Erythrodermic disease at presentation
>   - Rapid progression with involvement of large body areas
>   - Absence of inflammation
>   - Exaggerated inflammation (especially post initiation of therapy)
>   - Poor or partial response to standard dosing of conventional topical and systemic antifungals
>   - Persistent eczematous changes post-therapy
>   - Involvement of multiple family members
>   - Coexistent bacterial infections, e.g., furunculosis
>   - Frequent relapses/quick relapses
>   - Disabling itch (frequent nocturnal aggravation)
>   - Persistent itch after resolution
> - Signs of steroid abuse or irritant dermatitis
> - *Changes in the impact of disease*:
>   - High impact on quality of life indices
>   - Higher cost of therapy
>   - Longer duration of therapy (>6–8 weeks)
>   - Higher chances of treatment failure
>   - More family members/close contacts affected

Factors Affecting Changes in the Pattern of Tinea Infections

This recalcitrant nature of the disease has been attributed to various factors. If we see the epidemiological triad, these include host factors, agent factors, and pharmacologic factors.

Host Factors

Self-medication (suggested either by family member/friend or chemist) has been considered responsible for emergence of resistance against many antimicrobials. Dermatophytoses are no exception. This has directly as well as indirectly led to altered and difficult-to-treat tinea.

- Potent topical steroids (Schedule H drugs) are used rampantly due to easy over-the-counter availability in India due to poor implementation of control measures. They are economical as well as compared to topical antifungals. The patient's readiness to use them for symptomatic relief has been directly as well as indirectly responsible for altered presentation and recalcitrance of the disease.
- Use of tight, synthetic, and occlusive clothing provides an ideal environment for the fungus to flourish in a tropical climate like ours.
- Overcrowding and sharing of infected clothing promote spread of infection through fomites.
- Global warming with higher temperatures, prolonged summers, and more humidity predisposes to fungal infections.
- Often, there is a failure to address comorbid situations such as diabetes mellitus, obesity, and immunosuppression satisfactorily, resulting in poor treatment outcome.
- As the treatment duration is long and disease is not life threatening, there is nonadherence to the treatment schedule after initial relief.

Agent Factors

There has been a significant epidemiological shift regarding etiological agents. With the evaluation of emerging drug resistance and its molecular basis, the emergence of resistant species has also been recognized.

- The once common *Trichophyton rubrum* has been slowly outnumbered by *Trichophyton mentagrophytes,* which has better adaptability to the human body and survives longer on fomites outside the body. *T. mentagrophytes* infection is considered responsible for more widespread inflammatory lesions with pustulation.
- The incidence of primary drug resistance to terbinafine and fluconazole has been rising.

- *Trichophyton indotineae* is a newly identified species, isolated in near-epidemic proportions now, in a number of countries. It is identical to genotype VIII within the *T. mentagrophytes/T. interdigitale* species complex. It was described in 2019 by sequencing the *internal transcribed spacer* (ITS) region of ribosomal DNA. More than 10 ITS genotypes of *T. interdigitale* and *T. mentagrophytes* have been identified. Among these, *T. indotineae* seems to be the most problematic. It causes inflammatory, itchy, widespread disease affecting the groins, gluteal region, trunk, and face. It has been isolated from patients of all age groups and genders. It has been documented to have in-vitro genetic resistance to terbinafine (point mutations in the *squalene epoxidase* gene), translating to high in-vivo resistance.

Pharmacologic Factors

- The use of potent topical steroids or oral steroids/injectable steroids for superficial dermatophytosis is very rampant. It has been one of the most important factors responsible for the growing menace of superficial dermatophytosis. There are plenty of erratic and irrational steroid, antifungal, antibiotic combinations available as over-the-counter products that can be bought without prescription. The use of potent topical/injectable/oral steroids leads to an initial transient response and patient may feel symptomatically better. However, their uncontrolled use leads to grim and undesired consequences.
- Fungistatic nature of most of the antifungal drugs as well as their inappropriate/inadequate dosings is the practice that promotes resistance.
- Prolonged therapy with terbinafine and itraconazole, or even with topical antifungals, becomes expensive for the patients. This leads to noncompliance and inadequate treatment, further promoting resistance.
- Poor control of drug quality during production leads to a poor bioavailability of the active ingredient. It has often been seen that cheap medications may be of suboptimal quality as often economy is associated with poor efficacy.
- Many patients with extensive disease also have comorbidities such as diabetes mellitus, hypertension, or cardiac problems. They tend to be on polypharmacy leading to side effects/drug interactions. This often results in poor compliance or poor bioavailability.

CHANGING PATTERNS OF SUPERFICIAL DERMATOPHYTOSIS

The recalcitrant tinea infection often presents with atypical clinical presentations. These are detailed in the following text.

UNUSUALLY EXTENSIVE DISEASE

Tinea infections were conventionally limited to a part of the body. It has now become common to see involvement of multiple anatomic sites including axillae, groins, trunk, hands, feet, and nails in a single patient **(Figs. 1 to 3)**.

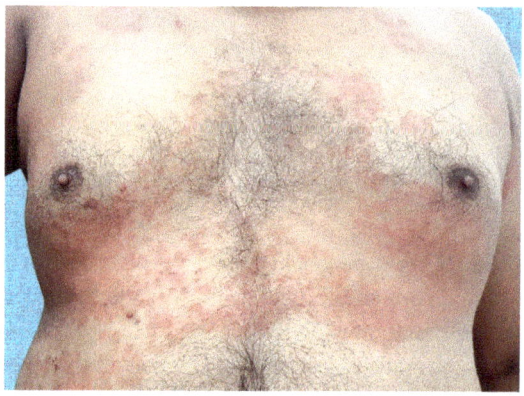

Fig. 1: Extensive tinea involving trunk and extending to axillae as well.

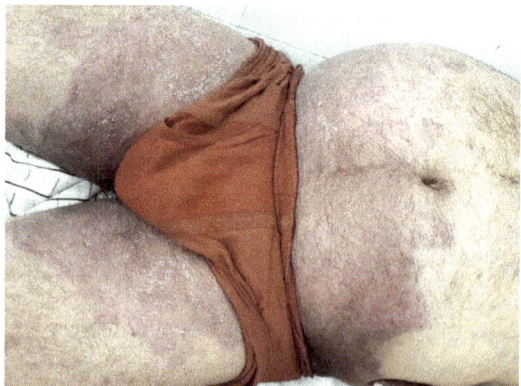

Fig. 2: Extensive tinea involving the lower abdomen up to the mid-thigh region. Both groins and genitalia were involved.

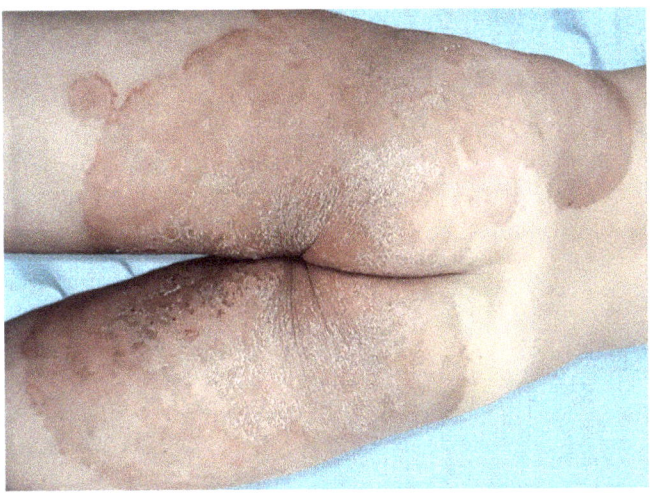

Fig. 3: Extensive tinea involving the trunk, buttocks, and legs (up to mid-thigh).

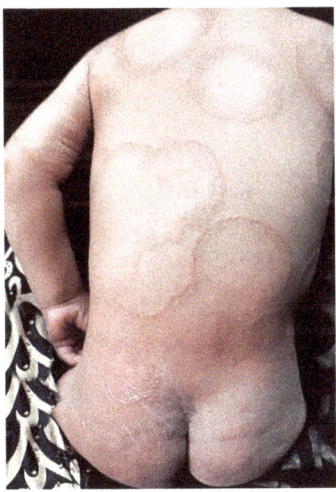

Fig. 4: Extensive tinea involving trunk in a 6-month-old infant.

OCCURRENCE IN INFANTS AND YOUNG CHILDREN

The presentation with extensive tinea lesions in small children is seen more often now. This is generally seen when either parents or close family members are involved and there is sharing of clothing **(Figs. 4 to 6)**. Even in children, the disease tends to be extensive and atypical.

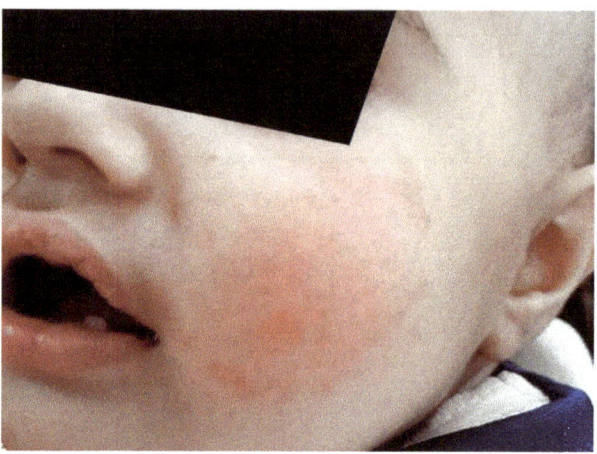

Fig. 5: Tinea faciei in a 3-month-old child.

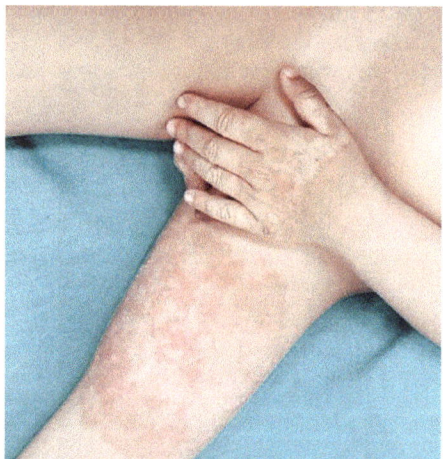

Fig. 6: Extensive tinea involving distinct areas of the body. There is involvement of groin (tinea cruris) up to the mid-thigh with limb extremity (tinea manuum) in a 2-year-old child.

Unusual Morphology (Tinea Incognito)

There is a higher incidence of difficult-to-recognize presentations and unusual morphologies. These include the following morphological presentations:
- *Tinea pseudoimbricata*: This clinically manifests as a "ring inside a ring" or "waves or rings" of tinea. This presentation generally results from topical steroid application **(Figs. 7 to 9)**.

CHAPTER 8: Recalcitrant Dermatophytosis

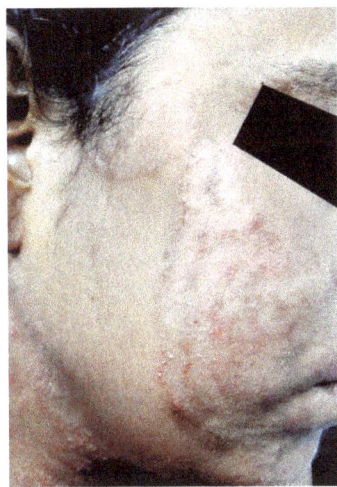

Fig. 7: Tinea pseudoimbricata involving face.

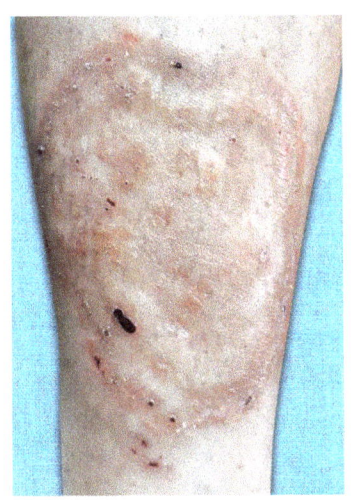

Fig. 8: Tinea pseudoimbricata involving the limbs.

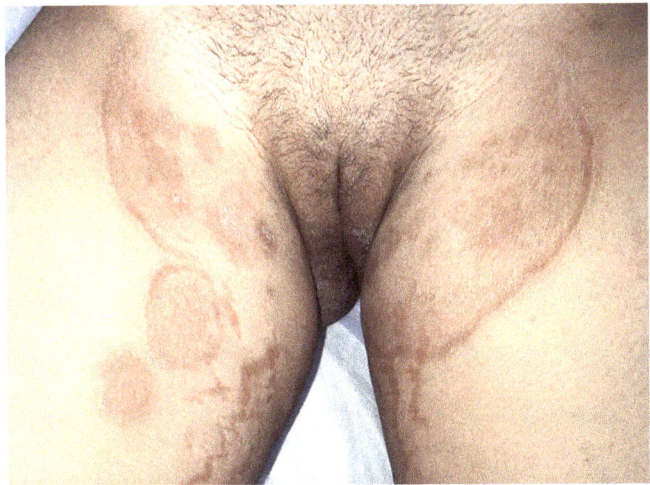

Fig. 9: Tinea pseudoimbricata in the groin area due to repeated steroid application.

- *Pustular tinea*: Pustular presentation is generally seen in patients with tinea, who were on prolonged steroid use (systemic or topical) and have suddenly stopped it **(Figs. 10 and 11)**. This withdrawal is associated with a pustular flare with intense itching.

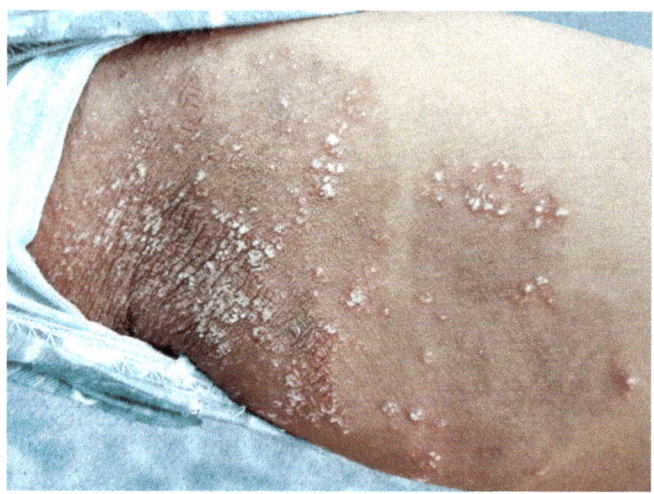

Fig. 10: Pustular tinea in a patient with prolonged steroid usage.

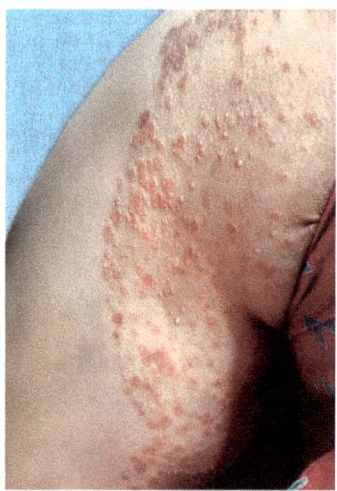

Fig. 11: Pustular and follicular inflammatory lesions. The modified tinea.

- *Tinea faciei*: Face was a less commonly seen area of involvement. However, it is much more commonly seen now. This could be related to the irrational use of topical steroid preparations on the face, which is common in desire of a fairer skin, for treatment of melasma, or for any facial pigmentation **(Figs. 12 to 16)**. This form of tinea is generally

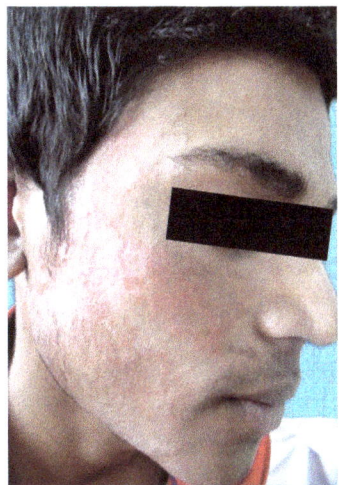

Fig. 12: Extensive tinea pseudoimbricata involving face.

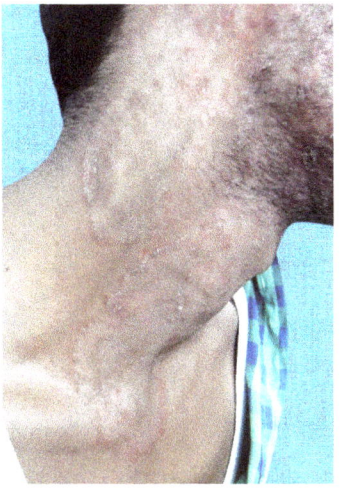

Fig. 13: Extensive tinea faciei extending up to the neck.

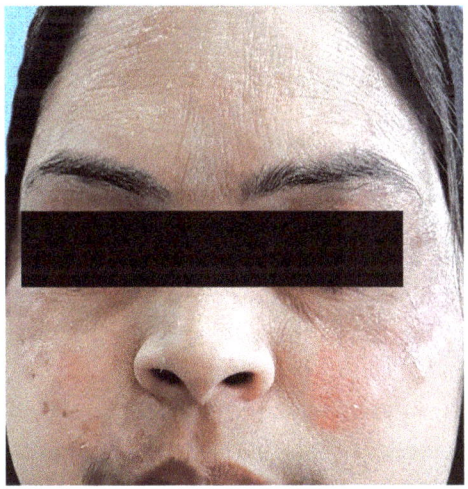

Fig. 14: Extensive tinea faciei involving almost the whole face, with indistinct margins.

accompanied by the involvement of vellus hair of sideburns. It necessitates systemic antifungal drug use.
- *Tinea auricularis*: Involvement of the external ear, with lesion extending up to the concha, is also seen now **(Fig. 17)**.

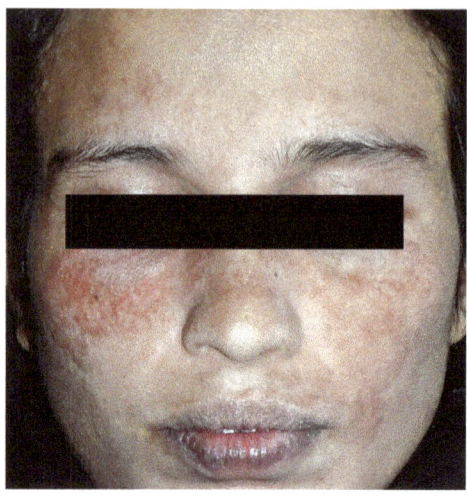

Fig. 15: Extensive bilaterally symmetrical tinea faciei with intense erythema, simulating a malar rash.

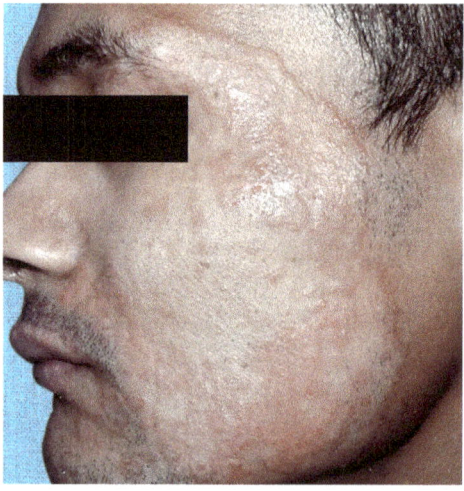

Fig. 16: Tinea faciei involving the whole central face, with extensive spread up to the sideburns.

- *Tinea of the scalp*: This is also an emerging modification, where extensive involvement of the scalp skin, extending on to the adjacent skin of forehead or the nape of the neck is seen. It tends to be noninflammatory. The extension of dermatophytosis to involve the terminal scalp hair even in adults necessitates prolonged systemic antifungal treatment **(Figs. 18 to 20)**.

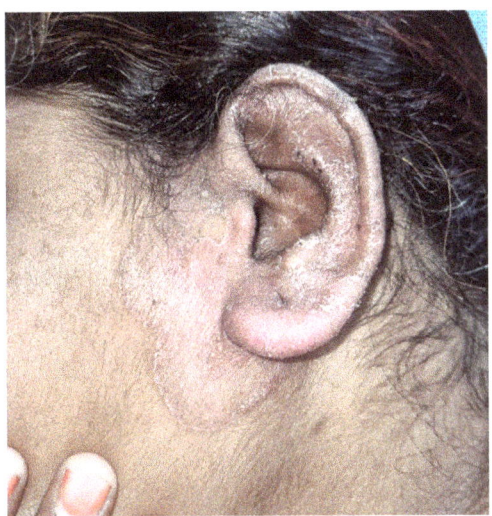

Fig. 17: Tinea auricularis.

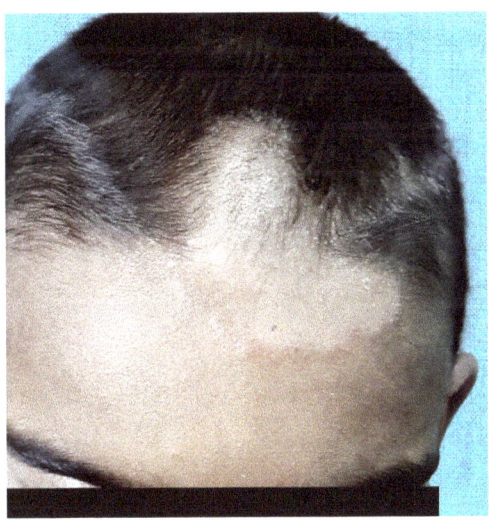

Fig. 18: Tinea of the scalp causing frontal hair loss. It is extending on to the forehead skin.

- *Diffuse scaly tinea with ill-defined margins*: The conventional well-defined margins of tinea corporis tend to be very ill-defined in patients using steroids. The lesions also have diffuse scaling. They may appear very dry or very eczematous in certain areas. Every suspected scaly

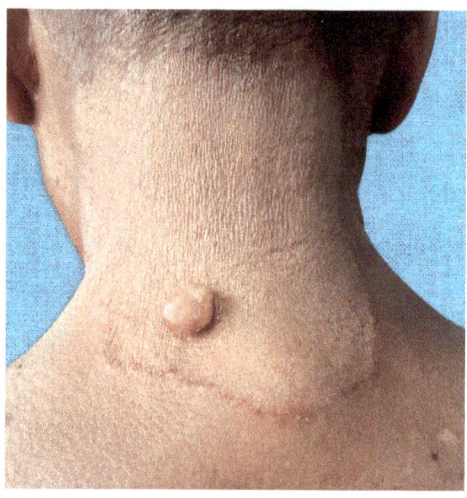

Fig. 19: Tinea of the posterior scalp with tinea corporis extending over the back of the neck.

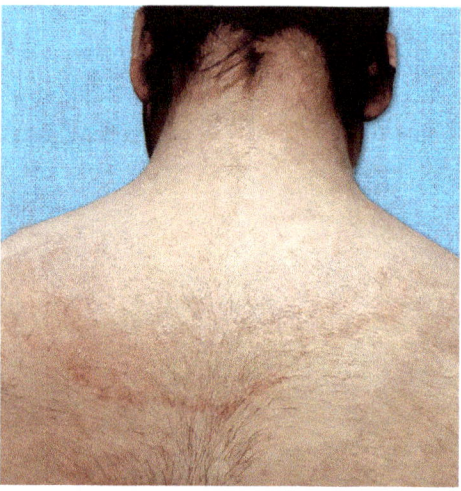

Fig. 20: Extensive involvement with tinea corporis that has contiguously extended to involve the scalp causing patchy hair loss.

lesion with margins (whether or not well-defined) with or without central clearing should be tested for fungal infection. This can be done with potassium hydroxide (KOH) scraping. This should be done before prescribing topical steroids **(Figs. 21 to 25)**.

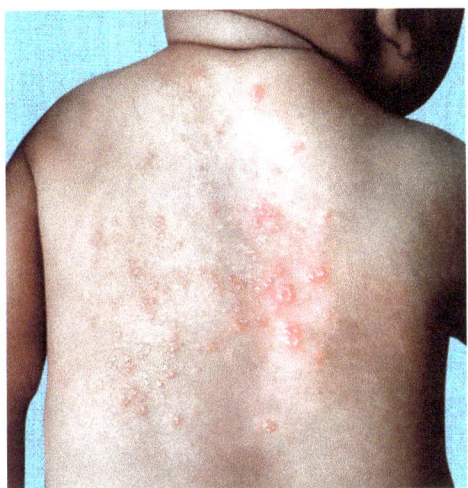

Fig. 21: Diffuse scaly tinea corporis in a young child. The lesion also has ill-defined margins. This presentation is commonly seen with steroid-modified tinea.

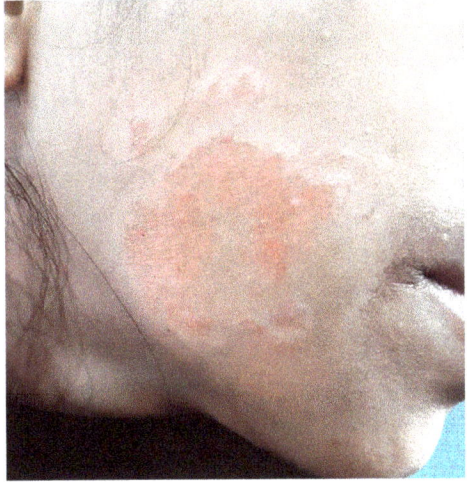

Fig. 22: Tinea faciei lesion with ill-defined margins. The erythema and scaling are secondary to topical steroid use.

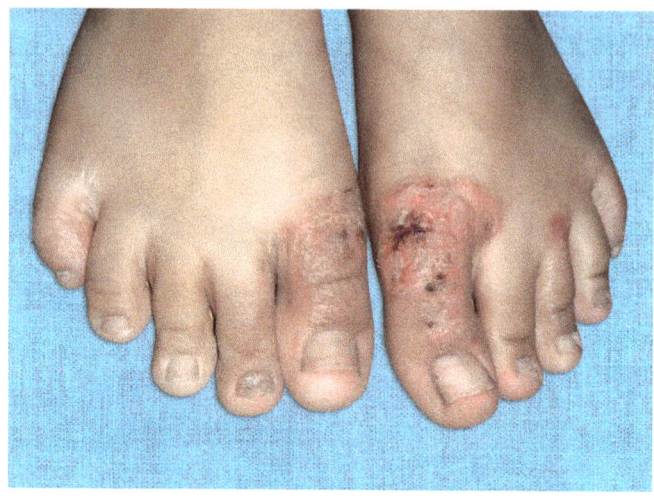

Fig. 23: Atypical symmetrical tinea pedis. The lesions appear very eczematous, but have a defined margin.

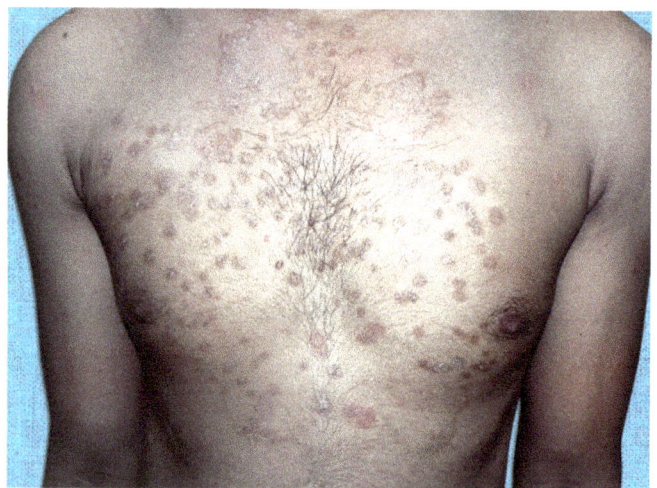

Fig. 24: Extensive truncal tinea corporis with numerous small lesions with well to ill-defined margins.

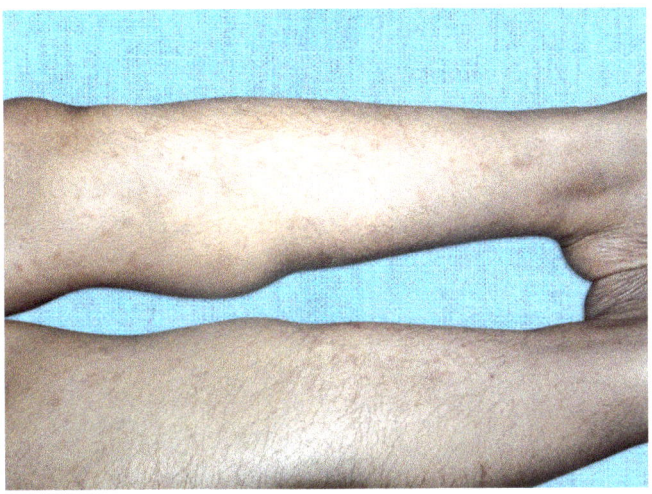

Fig. 25: Tinea corporis involving both legs with numerous, small, scaly lesions. The condition is highly steroid modified.

- *Tinea of vellus hair*: This entity is being increasingly recognized, with more effective diagnostic techniques and closer examination. A clinical recognition of involvement of vellus hair, even in seemingly localized tinea, has made us more aware toward the need for systemic therapy in such cases. Tinea of vellus hair may be responsible for relapse and poor treatment response in a large number of cases. It can be documented using a dermatoscope as well as KOH mount.
- *Tinea in immune-compromised districts*: An aberration in the immune control of a localized area of skin, affected by another disease process, is known as an immunocompromised district. There has been an increasing recognition of atypical tinea lesions appearing secondarily over such areas **(Fig. 26)**. These include areas such as amputation stumps, surgical incision sites, tattooed skin, areas with resolved tinea lesions, apart from areas with topical steroid application. Immune-mediated dermatoses such as vitiligo and lichen planus are also known to develop preferentially at the sites of tinea corporis.

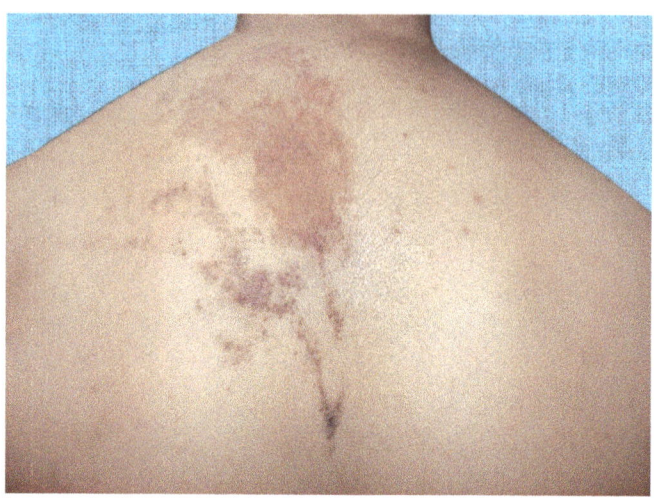

Fig. 26: Tinea corporis localizing to areas with segmental lichen planus on the back of a young male.

SIGNS OF CORTICOSTEROID OR IRRITANT USE

Familiarity with signs and stigmata of steroid abuse as well-repeated use of irritants is important to recognize for the treating physician.

- Abuse of potent topical steroid is associated with striae and hypopigmentation. Striae mostly occur early with potent steroid-containing combinations **(Fig. 27)**. They are most pronounced in the flexures including axillae and thighs. Initial erythematous phase (striae rubra) is followed by whitish striae (striae alba).
- Occasional ulceration may be seen due to extreme thinning of skin, induced by steroids **(Figs. 28 and 29)**. These ulcers tend to become secondarily infected. Striae may assume a pseudoedematous appearance at times. Patients may deny continued usage; however, depot effect of steroids ensures continued ulceration.
- Red scrotum syndrome (persistent scrotal erythema) is seen in some patients applying fixed-dose combinations containing topical steroids **(Fig. 29)**.
- Lesional and perilesional hypopigmentation develops within 3-4 weeks. It may be accompanied by atrophy and telangiectasia. It is also seen with intralesional steroid injections, especially in a linear pattern.

CHAPTER 8: Recalcitrant Dermatophytosis

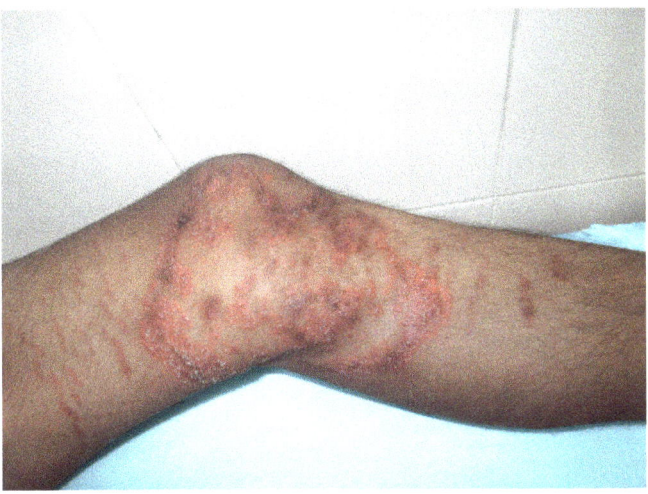

Fig. 27: Inflamed lesion of tinea corporis in a male with chronic steroid use as evidenced by extensive striae and erythema.

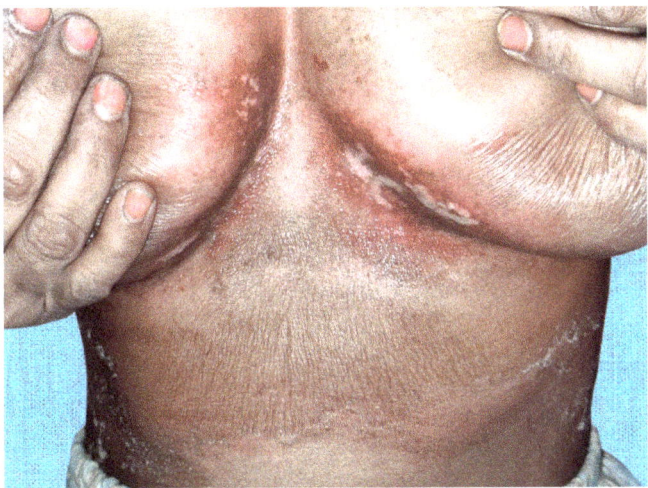

Fig. 28: An old lady with extensive tinea corporis, steroid induced striae, thinning of skin, ulceration of skin and secondary bacterial infection in the inframammary area.

- Bacteria can concomitantly infect and complicate tinea lesions. This is due to local immunosuppression due to topical steroids.
- Signs of irritant dermatitis include erythema, brownish discoloration, scaling, and exfoliation. These may be seen over and around infected

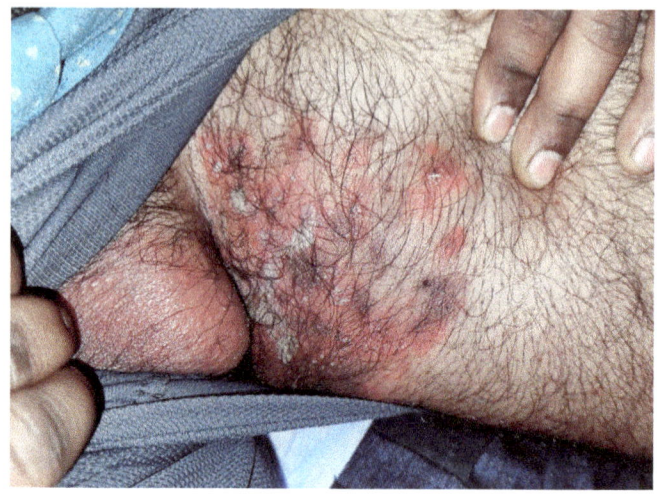

Fig. 29: Inflamed lesion of tinea cruris with secondary ulceration, infection, and red scrotal skin.

sites and are commonly seen due to use of home remedies including crushed plant extracts or lotions, and over-the-counter preparations containing salicylic acid, sulfur, etc. Associated symptoms include burning, pain, and tenderness.
- Iatrogenic Cushing's syndrome may be seen in patients with extensive tinea, and is suggestive of a possibility of systemic steroid intake over a long period of time. These include higher weight, truncal obesity, striking striae, acneiform eruption, hypertrichosis, and hirsutism.

IMPACT OF RECALCITRANT DERMATOPHYTOSIS

The disease behaves like other chronic and recurrent disorders and has a significant bearing on the quality of life, emotions, and personal relationships of the patients. It may be responsible for feelings of hopelessness, shame and anger, even suicidal ideation.

Also, the disease preferentially affects people from lower socioeconomic strata, and may often affect multiple family members. It also requires prolonged antifungal therapy. All this adds up to a significant financial burden. This is turn may contribute to poor compliance and consequently poor efficacy.

CHAPTER 9

Tinea Capitis

INTRODUCTION

Dermatophytic infection of the scalp hair follicles is known as tinea capitis. It is also known as tinea tonsurans. It mostly affects children in the preadolescent age group, though rarely adults can also develop this infection. There is no gender predilection. The infection is common in India, Africa, and certain urban areas of North, Central, and South America. It commonly affects school-going children and households with overcrowding.

Tinea capitis is a worldwide problem. The predominant species causing tinea capitis varies from region to region and time to time. The most common species worldwide is *Microsporum canis*, though there has been an increase in the prevalence of *Trichophyton tonsurans* prevalence, especially in the United States and in western Europe. The incidence of tinea capitis in India varies from 0.5 to 10%. Here, *Trichophyton violaceum* is the most common species isolated.

ETIOPATHOGENESIS

All dermatophytic molds are known to invade the hair shaft except for three species—*Trichophyton concentricum*, *Trichophyton mentagrophytes var. interdigitale* and *Epidermophyton floccosum*. Thus, tinea capitis can be potentially caused by all dermatophytes except these.

The infection starts when arthroconidia circulating in the air get trapped into the scalp hair and start invading the scalp skin at the level of stratum corneum. The incubation period is approximately 3 weeks. From there, three main patterns of hair shaft invasion by the dermatophytic molds have been described. These include *ectothrix pattern* where the fungus penetrates at the midfollicular level of a mid- to-late anagen phase of hair follicle and grows downward toward the hair bulb until the upper border of keratinized zone. At this zone, also known as Adamson's fringe, the fungus multiplies in equilibrium with the rate of keratinization, thus invading the newly keratinized cells. There are two types of ectothrix spores. The small-spored ectothrix is seen with *Microsporum canis, Microsporum audouinii, Microsporum equinum,* or *Microsporum ferrugineum* species mainly. Secondary extrapilary hyphae grow out in a tortuous manner and then segment into a mass of small arthroconidias of size 2–3 μm. This type shows green fluorescence under Wood's lamp. The large-spored ectothrix pattern is a result of infection with *T. mentagrophytes var. mentagrophytes, Trichophyton verrucosum, Microsporum gypseum,* and *Microsporum fulvum.* Here, the primary straight extrapilary hyphae break into chains of large arthroconidia of size 5–8 μm on the surface of hair follicle and there is no fluorescence on Wood's lamp examination.

The second pattern is the *endothrix pattern.* Here, the penetration is in a manner similar to ectothrix, but there is intrapilary extension. The hyphae of *T. tonsurans* and *T. violaceum* species break into multiple large arthroconidia (8–10 μm) inside the hair shaft making it weak and fragile. As a result, the hair follicle breaks at the level of skin surface leaving behind black dots while the cortex remains intact.

The third pattern is known as *favus.* It is caused by *Trichophyton schoenleinii.* The intrapilary hyphae, rather than breaking up into arthroconidia, remain intact inside the hair shaft. As a result, the hair grows and attains normal length unlike endothrix. However, the tunnels formed inside the hair follicle appear as air spaces under KOH mount.

CLINICAL FEATURES

The clinical presentation of tinea capitis varies greatly, depending on the causative species, the type of hair invasion, and the level of host resistance. Tinea capitis appearance may vary from noninflammatory types like gray patch to severe inflammatory variants like kerion. The inflammatory variants may have associated cervical or occipital lymphadenopathy. However, a great degree of overlap and coexistence of different patterns in the same patient may occur. The common clinical presentation in all forms is partial hair loss, which is noncicatricial but may be cicatricial in many cases.

- *Gray patch or noninflammatory tinea capitis* is generally associated with *Microsporum audouinii or Microsporum ferrugenium* infection, which produce a small-spored ectothrix type of penetration. It is typically seen in the form of well-circumscribed round patches of noncicatricial alopecia, with multiple broken stumps of gray, lusterless hair and mild scaling **(Fig. 1)**. The arthroconidia coating the hair give rise to the gray appearance. *M. canis* may produce a similar picture albeit with a little more inflammation.
- *Black dot tinea capitis* is caused by species like *T. tonsurans, T. violaceum,* and *Trichophyton soudanense,* which produce an endothrix pattern of invasion. It is characterized by grouped black dots (swollen hair shafts, broken at the scalp surface) associated with diffuse scaling **(Fig. 2)**. The inflammation may vary from mild scaling to frank pustule formation. More inflammation is generally associated with zoophilic species. The lesions are usually multiple and have angulated borders unlike those of gray patch tinea capitis.
- *Inflammatory tinea capitis* is usually seen in cases with infection with zoophilic species like *T. mentagrophytes var. mentagrophytes* and *T. verrucosum.* It is also associated with geophilic species like *M. gypseum.* Inflammatory tinea capitis is characterized by a hypersensitivity response to the invading fungus. The clinical presentations may vary from follicular pustules **(Fig. 3)** to frank

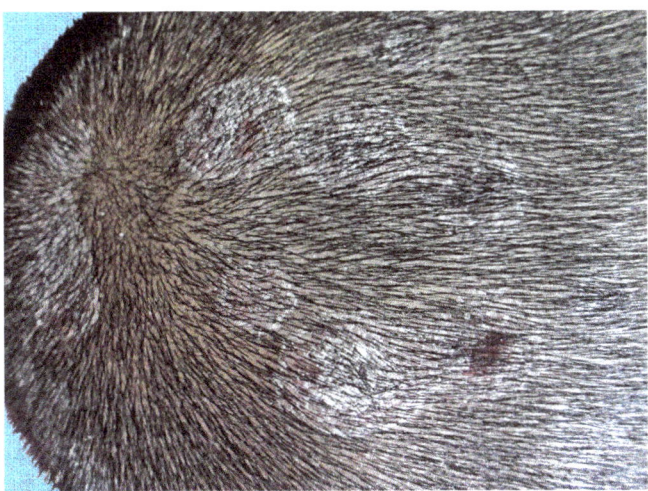

Fig. 1: Gray patch tinea capitis.

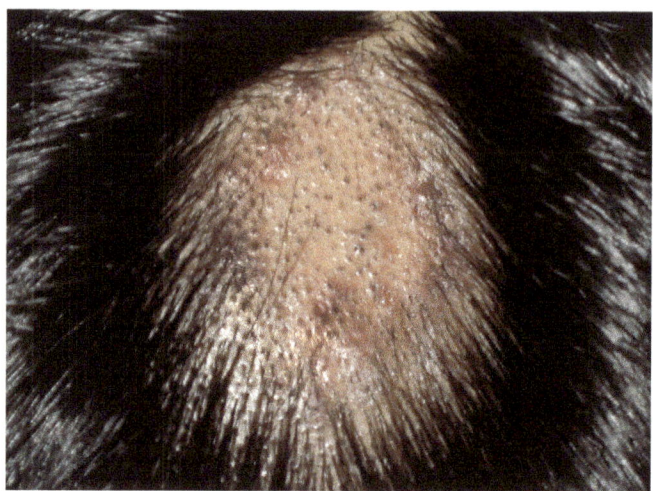

Fig. 2: Black dot tinea capitis.

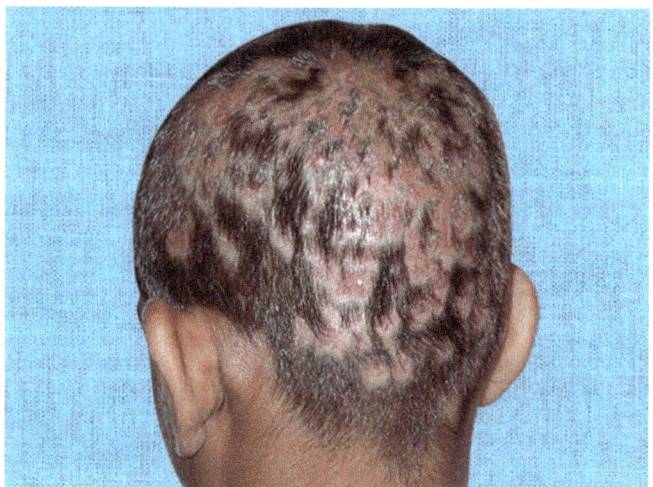

Fig. 3: Inflammatory tinea capitis.

kerion formation (an inflammatory, painful boggy swelling studded with follicular pustules) along with associated lymphadenopathy **(Fig. 4)**. Although self-resolution may occur in some cases, scarring is the usual outcome, causing cicatricial alopecia. The affected patients may also develop an id eruption.

CHAPTER 9: Tinea Capitis

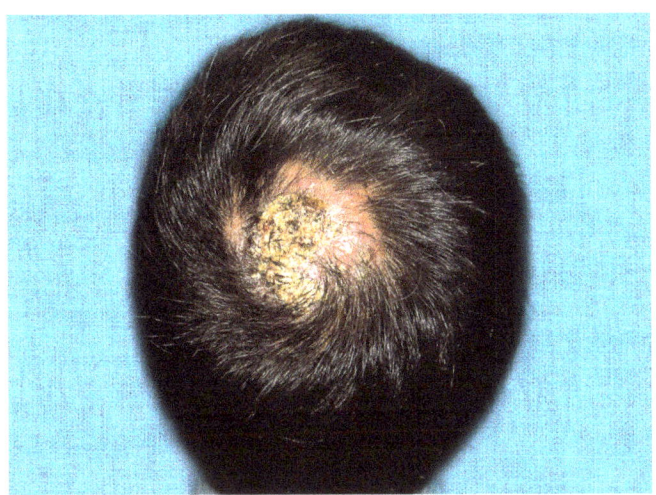

Fig. 4: Kerion.

- *Favus* is a type of tinea capitis, caused by the species *T. schoenleinii*. Cases occur sporadically in the South African countries, Middle East, and Pakistan. It is a long-standing infection, which may extend over many years. It is characterized by yellow colored cup-shaped scutulum around the hair follicles, which may become confluent to form yellow crusts. The infection is usually chronic with little tendency for self-resolution and with the risk of development of cicatricial alopecia.

DIFFERENTIAL DIAGNOSIS

The differential diagnoses for tinea capitis are summarized in **Box 1**.

BOX 1	Differential diagnosis of tinea capitis.
• Seborrheic dermatitis • Psoriasis • Atopic dermatitis • Alopecia areata	• Trichotillomania • Bacterial folliculitis or impetigo • Folliculitis decalvans

CHAPTER 10

Onychomycosis

INTRODUCTION

Onychomycosis refers to fungal infection of the nail unit. It accounts for up to 50% of dystrophic nails. Tinea unguium refers to onychomycosis caused by dermatophytes. Being a complex appendage, the nail offers unique challenges to fungi and also manifests variable features giving rise to distinctive clinical types of onychomycosis.

Onychomycosis is common infection (community prevalence of 3–5%, even up to 26%). Its incidence is highly variable across the world depending on socioeconomic and cultural factors. Up to 30% of patients with dermatophytosis of skin are likely to have onychomycosis.

ETIOPATHOGENESIS

A variety of fungi have been implicated as causative of onychomycosis. A large European study (Achilles foot project) evaluating diseased feet and nails (80,396 patients) found the following results in cases with onychomycosis:
- Tinea unguium or onychomycosis caused by dermatophytes was the most common (68% cases).
- Candidal onychomycosis accounted for 11% cases.
- Nondermatophyte mould infection (NDM onychomycosis) also accounted for 11% cases.
- No mycological growth was seen in 10.9% cases, while mixed infections were seen in 0.1% cases.
  Few important causative species are outlined in **Table 1**.

TABLE 1: Important causative species isolated in cases with onychomycosis.		
Dermatophytes	**Yeasts**	**Nondermatophyte moulds**
Trichophyton rubrum (most common cause); *Trichophyton mentagrophytes* var. *interdigitale*; *Epidermophyton floccosum*; *Trichophyton verrucosum*; *Microsporum* species	*Candida albicans*; *C. parapsilosis*; *C. krusei*; *C. tropicalis*	*Aspergillus* species (niger/fumigatus/flavus); *Scopulariopsis brevicaulis*; *Scytalidium dimidiatum*; *Acremonium* species; *Alternaria* species; *Neoscytalidium* species; *Fusarium* species.

CLINICAL FEATURES

The following main clinical types **(Table 2)** of onychomycosis are recognized: Distal and lateral subungual onychomycosis (DLSO) **(Fig. 1)**, proximal subungual onychomycosis (PSO) **(Fig. 2)**, superficial onychomycosis (SO) **(Fig. 3)**, and endonyx onychomycosis **(Fig. 4)**. Additional variants include total dystrophic onychomycosis (TDO) **(Fig. 5)**, mixed patterns (may be seen in some cases), and secondary onychomycosis, which is the infection of already traumatized or diseased nail plate like psoriatic nails **(Fig. 6)**. TDO is the result of severe nail infection, involving the whole thickness of the nail pate, nail bed, and nail matrix (with the nail becoming thickened and crumbling down).

TINEA UNGUIUM

Invasion of the nail plate by dermatophytes is known as tinea unguium. It is more common in adults, especially males, due to their propensity to trauma related to occupation, sports, or leisure activities.

Etiopathogenesis

The most common dermatophytes responsible for nail plate invasion are *Trichophyton rubrum* (more than half of cases), *Trichophyton mentagrophytes var. interdigitale* (both accounting for up to 90% cases), and *Epidermophyton floccosum* (1.2%). Dermatophytes are keratinophiles; thus, they affect keratin-rich nail plate structure. Fungal pathogenicity varies with species, with *Trichophyton mentagrophyte*s being considered a more active destroyer than *T. rubrum*.

SECTION 2: Dermatophytosis

TABLE 2: Different clinical types of onychomycosis.

Clinical type	Most common species	Site of invasion	Clinical features	Special considerations
Distal and lateral subungual onychomycosis (DLSO) **(Fig. 1)**	*Trichophyton rubrum*	Hyponychium and distal nail bed, progresses proximally	Thickening and yellow or brown discoloration of nail plate, distal onycholysis, and subungual hyperkeratosis	• Most common clinical type • Toenails more commonly affected than finger nails • Usually accompanied with tinea pedis and tinea manuum
Proximal subungual onychomycosis (PSO) **(Fig. 2)**	• *Trichophyton rubrum* • *Trichophyton menignii*	Proximal nail fold	Proximal onycholysis, subungual hyperkeratosis, and destruction of the proximal nail plate	• AIDS patients • Periungual inflammation can also occur
Superficial white onychomycosis (SWO) **(Fig. 3)**	*Trichophyton mentagrophytes var. interdigitale*	Dorsal surface of nail plate	Patches of pseudoleukonychia from which powdery material can be scraped off	• Toenails more commonly affected than the finger nails • AIDS patients • Rare variant • May be caused by NDM like *Acremonium, Aspergillus, Fusarium*
Endonyx onychomycosis (EO) **(Fig. 4)**	*Trichophyton soudanense, Trichophyton violaceum*	Nail plate, growing between the lamellas	Milky white patches with pits. Nail plate surface and bed remains normal	

(AIDS: acquired immunodeficiency syndrome; NDM: nondermatophytic mould)

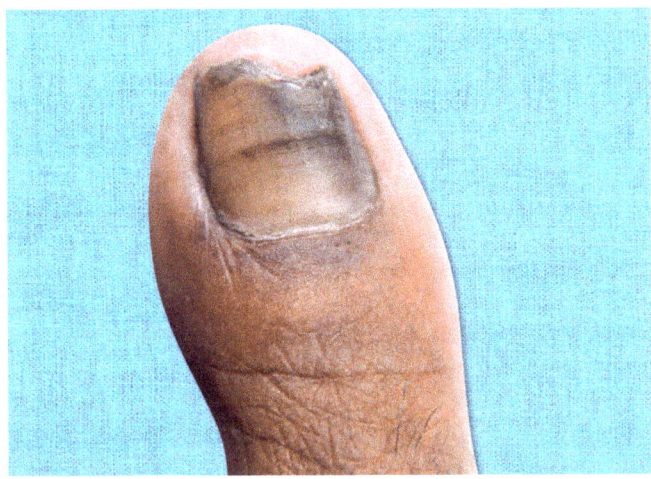

Fig. 1: Distal and lateral subungual onychomycosis involving the thumb nail.

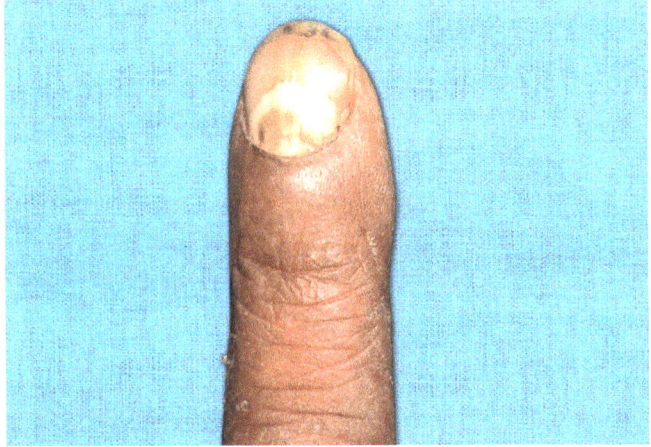

Fig. 2: Proximal subungual onychomycosis.

Differential Diagnosis

The differential diagnoses for tinea unguium are summarized in **Table 3**. The clinical presentation of tinea unguium may closely mimic a myriad of nail pathologies. It is often difficult to make a distinction on clinical grounds alone. Apart from this, tinea unguium has to be differentiated from onychomycosis caused by *Candida* and nondermatophytic moulds (NDMs).

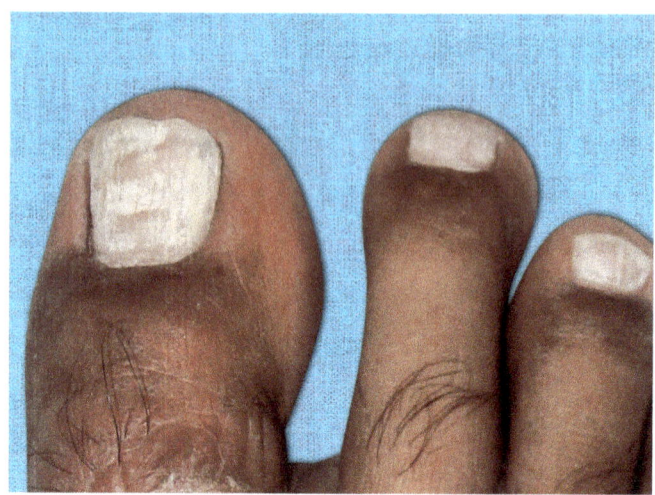

Fig. 3: Superficial white onychomycosis. Note the rough nail plate.

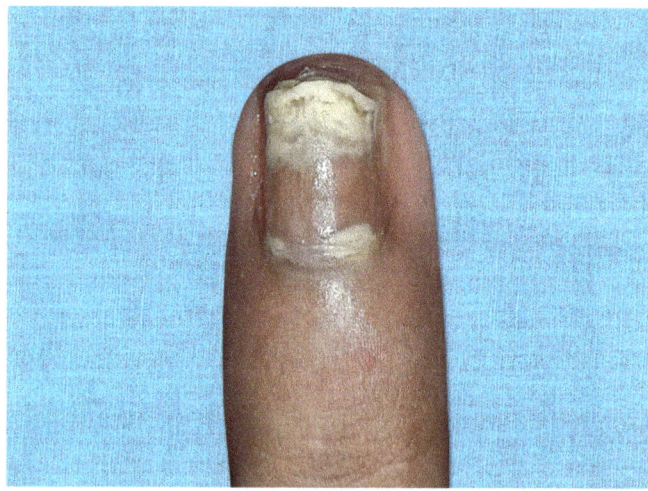

Fig. 4: Endonyx onychomycosis. Note the uninvolved nail bed and thickened and discolored nail plate with smooth surface.

Candidal Onychomycosis

The most common clinical presentation of onychomycosis caused by *Candida* species is as DLSO. Primary yeast onychomycosis (*Candida* species) is rare, seen only in those with immunosuppression. More commonly, *Candida* is a secondary invader.

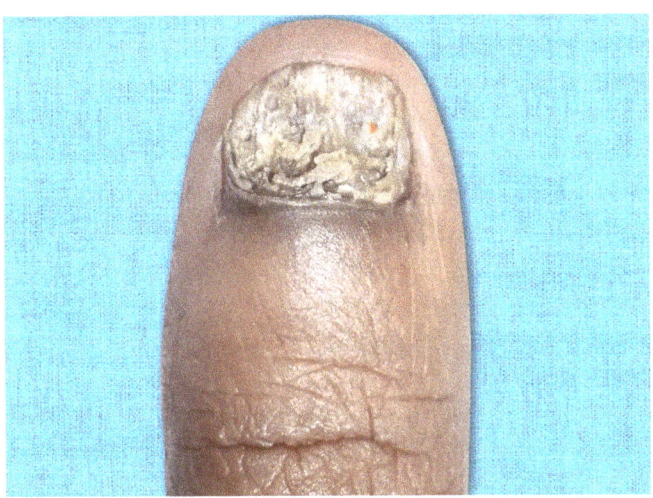

Fig. 5: Total dystrophic onychomycosis.

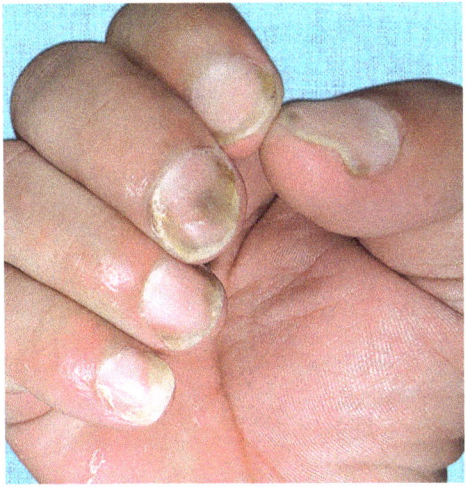

Fig. 6: Fungal infection of psoriatic nails. Distal onycholysis with the characteristic erythematous border can be appreciated.

This distal and lateral onycholysis is associated with subungual hyperkeratosis in addition to an evidence of paronychia **(Fig. 7)**. In few cases, there may be presence of only erosions of lateral and distal nail plates along with paronychia.

SECTION 2: Dermatophytosis

TABLE 3: Differential diagnosis of tinea unguium.

Disease	Clinical clues
Nail psoriasis	Fine pits, oil drop sign, splinter hemorrhages, multiple nail involvement
Chronic eczema	Irregular course pits with proximal nail fold involvement
Nail lichen planus	Thinning of the nail plate, nail splitting, longitudinal ridges
Pachyonychia congenita	Can be late onset and difficult to distinguish
Congenital or acquired leukonychia	History generally provides the clue
NDM onychomycosis	Periungual inflammation, brownish discoloration of nail plate
Candidal onychomycosis	Proximal nail fold swelling, Beau's lines

(NDM: nondermatophytic mould)

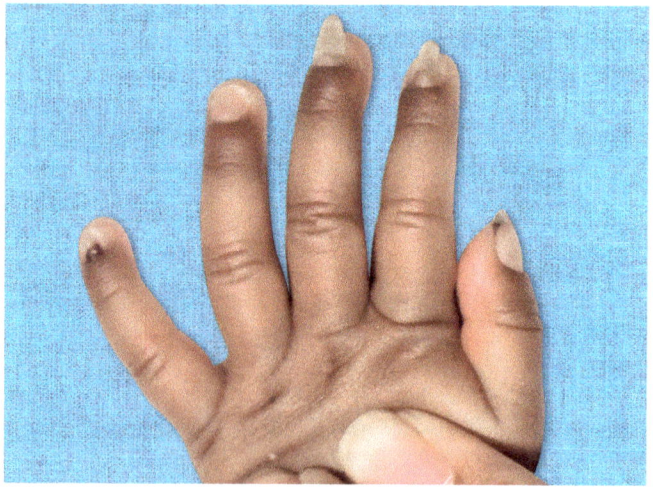

Fig. 7: Candidal onychomycosis in a young child.

NONDERMATOPHYTE MOULD INFECTIONS

Nondermatophyte moulds are responsible for nail infections mostly. They account for 1.5-11% of all onychomycosis as per various studies. NDMs can be primary pathogens or may be contaminants and secondary pathogens. NDM onychomycosis is becoming more common worldwide, accounting for 10% or more cases.

Nondermatophyte moulds are filamentous fungi, commonly found in nature as soil saprophytes and plant pathogens. The commonly isolated species are *Scopulariopsis brevicaulis, Aspergillus, Fusarium, Onychocola canadensis*, and *Scytalidium*. They affect the toenails mainly.

Usually, previously abnormal nails are affected as NDMs, as they generally do not infect previously normal nails unlike dermatophytes. Suggested predisposing factors include increasing age, immunosuppression, poor peripheral circulation, peripheral neuropathy, and trauma. Most of these molds are ubiquitous in the environment; hence, their isolation in fungal cultures from suspected nails should not by itself be considered as a proof of causation. Mostly, these are contaminants in fungal culture. They are considered pathogenic only if the following criteria are satisfied:
- Nail abnormalities are consistent with a diagnosis of NDM onychomycosis
- A positive direct microscopic examination visualizing fungal elements within the nail keratin
- Failure to isolate any dermatophyte species in fungal culture
- Growth of more than five colonies of the same mould in at least two consecutive nail samples

The clinical features of NDM onychomycosis are quite similar to dermatophyte onychomycosis. However, there are certain subtle differences in presentation. Thes include, the presence of periungual inflammation, brown discoloration of nail plate, and absence of concomitant skin involvement or tinea pedis.

Clinical clues toward possible causative fungus responsible for onychomycosis
- *T. rubrum* is the most common pathogen in distal lateral subungual onychomycosis.

- Proximal subungual onychomycosis due to *T. rubrum* infection is typical in immune-suppressed patients.
- Proximal subungual onychomycosis with periungual inflammation is usually caused by molds.
- White superficial onychomycosis is usually caused by *T. mentagrophytes*.
- NDMs cause deep white superficial onychomycosis.
- *Candida albicans* nail infection is observed in premature children, immune-compromised patients, and persons with chronic mucocutaneous candidiasis.

SECTION 3

Diagnosis of Dermatophytosis

Chapter 11: Dermatoscopy (Skin, Hair, and Nail) and Bedside Diagnosis of Dermatophytosis

Chapter 12: Laboratory Diagnosis

CHAPTER 11

Dermatoscopy (Skin, Hair, and Nail) and Bedside Diagnosis of Dermatophytosis

INTRODUCTION

Superficial dermatophytoses are the ones most commonly encountered. Herein, the infection remains confined to stratum corneum of skin, hair, or nails. The superficial mycoses, especially dermatophytosis, have assumed almost epidemic proportions of late. Due to their increasing incidence, altered behavior, newer presentation patterns, and refractoriness to routine treatment options, it is imperative that medical practitioners are made aware of this growing menace. It is important to learn to recognize it and treat it effectively while at the same time preventing transmission in the community.

BEDSIDE DIAGNOSIS OF SUPERFICIAL DERMATOPHYTOSES

Many cutaneous disorders can masquerade the superficial mycoses. There is a wide list of differentials as discussed with the above entities. Also, with rapid changes in clinical presentation and many confusing presentations, it becomes important to confirm diagnosis by various methods before starting the patients on prolonged antifungal therapy. The bedside diagnostic tests include examination with a dermatoscope as well as with Wood's lamp. Laboratory confirmation is based on direct microscopy, fungal culture, and histopathology.

Sampling Techniques

Bedside collection of adequate samples is the benchmark for the success of laboratory-based diagnosis. The results of the laboratory tests depend on the adequacy of the samples collected; hence, it is important to take samples properly to avoid false-negative results. The sampling techniques for various sites are summarized in **Table 1**. The specimen thus collected can be examined by direct microscopy, can be transported in a dry folded piece of paper for fungal isolation, or sent in formalin for histopathologic examination. It is important to avoid moisture to prevent rapid multiplication of bacteria.

Wood's Lamp Examination

Wood's lamp is a simple handy tool which is useful in diagnosing some superficial fungal infections including tinea capitis and pityriasis versicolor. Wood's lamp emits ultraviolet (UV)-A light and is fitted with a filter composed of barium silicate and 9% nickel oxide **(Fig. 1)**.

TABLE 1: Sampling techniques when a superficial fungal infection is suspected.	
Skin	The blunt end of the clean scalpel blade can be used to scrape the scales from the border of the lesion
Hair	In tinea capitis, the hair should be plucked with the forceps. Skin scrapings can also be taken from scalp in case of gray patch
Nail (finger and toe nails should be sampled if both are affected)	The hyperkeratotic nail bed can be scraped off with the blunt end of a disposable scalpel blade. The whole thickness of the nail plate can also be taken with the help of nail clipper

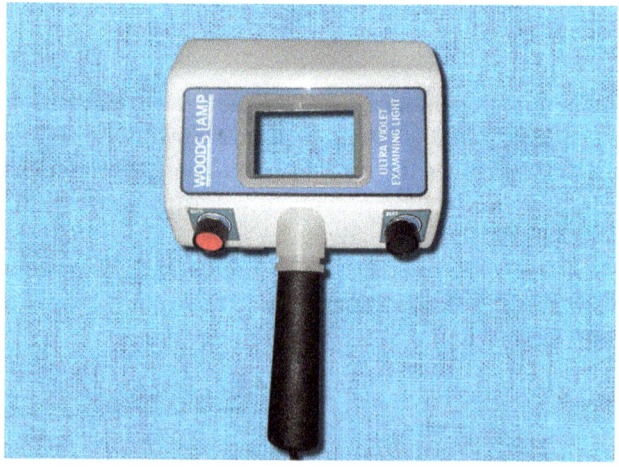

Fig. 1: Wood's lamp commonly used in dermatology clinics.

Fluorescence of tissues occurs when Wood's (UV) light is absorbed and radiation of a longer wavelength, usually visible light, is emitted. Small spored ectothrix infection caused by *Microsporum canis* and *Microsporum audouinii* produces brilliant green fluorescence under Wood's lamp. The causative agent of favus, *Trichophyton schonleinii*, can also produce pale green fluorescence. Similarly, pityriasis versicolor shows pale yellow to white fluorescence.

Dermatoscopy

Dermatoscopy is examination of skin and its appendages with a dermatoscope, which is an instrument with standard magnifying optics and a transilluminating light source. It allows noninvasive, in vivo, subsurface visualization of various skin disorders. Dermatoscopy is the standard of care around the world and is now becoming increasingly popular and of diagnostic value, with many more indications being explored.

Among the existing diagnostic modalities for superficial fungal infections, there are various constraints in the diagnostic output. This could be because of their complexity, time-consuming nature, lack of trained personnel, lack of laboratory support in many areas, and poor diagnostic efficacy even when this is provided. Hence, the role of dermoscopy assumes even greater importance.

Dermoscopy is a useful point-of-care test for tinea diagnosis. As compared to other point-of-care tests, i.e., direct microscopy, much lesser studies are available. However, it offers several advantages as it enables rapid, noninvasive, in vivo observation of fungal invasion. It can help identify suspect hair/nail for sampling. It can identify high-risk contacts as well as steroid-modified cases.

Tinea Capitis

Dermatophyte scalp infection is suggested by the presence of comma hair, corkscrew hair, zigzag hair, morse code/bar code hair, black dots, and dystrophic hair. These changes in tinea capitis are the most well studied, and there are comparative studies available evaluating the sensitivity and specificity of these findings in ruling out other causes of noncicatricial hair loss. Other features include the presence of erythema (as a background) or even in the form of elongated blood vessels. Scarring alopecia with tinea capitis is characterized by loss of follicular ostia and fibrosis. The lesions also show scaling which can be in the form of perifollicular scale or pilar casts. Presence of yellow dots may be seen in noncicatricial cases **(Figs. 2 to 7)**. Dermoscopic (trichoscopic) findings in tinea capitis are summarized in **Table 2**.

Onychomycosis

Dermatophyte nail infection is also well studied and evaluated with dermoscopy. Salient dermatoscopic features include onycholysis

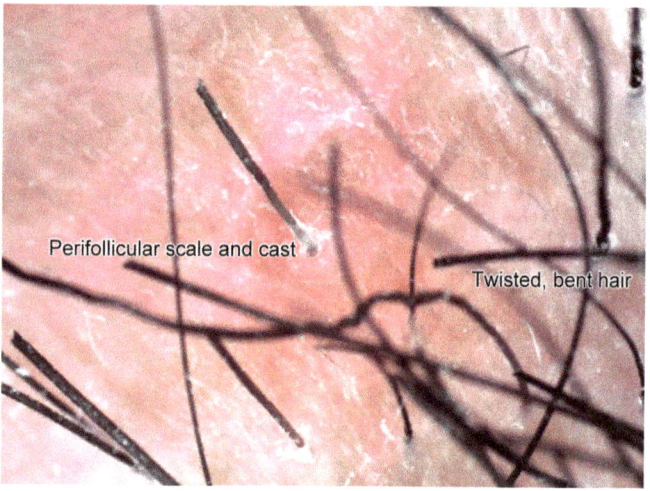

Fig. 2: Dermatoscopic image showing perifollicular scale along with twisted and bent hair.

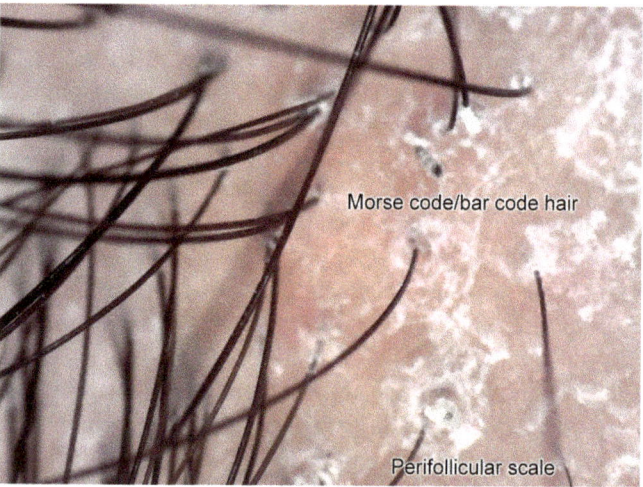

Fig. 3: Dermatoscopic image showing a single Morse code hair.

with jagged proximal edges, "spikes" within onycholytic nail plate, chromonychia (white, yellow, orange, brown color) leading to longitudinal striae (Aurora Borealis pattern), subungual "ruin" appearance, and a yellow orange nail plate **(Figs. 8 to 11)**. Dermoscopic (onychoscopic) findings in onychomycosis are summarized in **Table 3**.

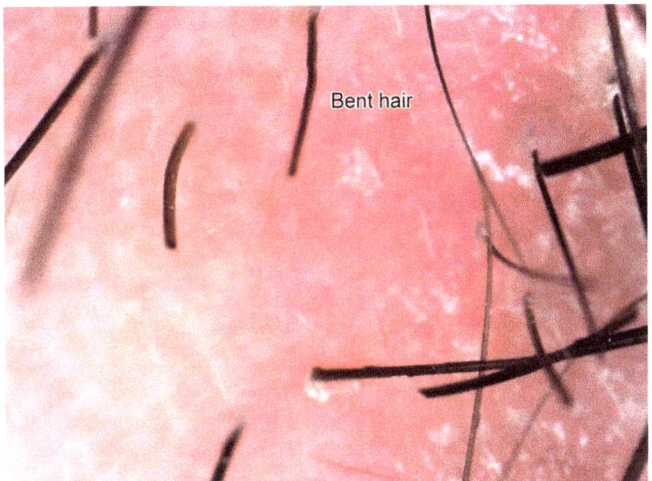

Fig. 4: Dermatoscopic image showing a bent hair.

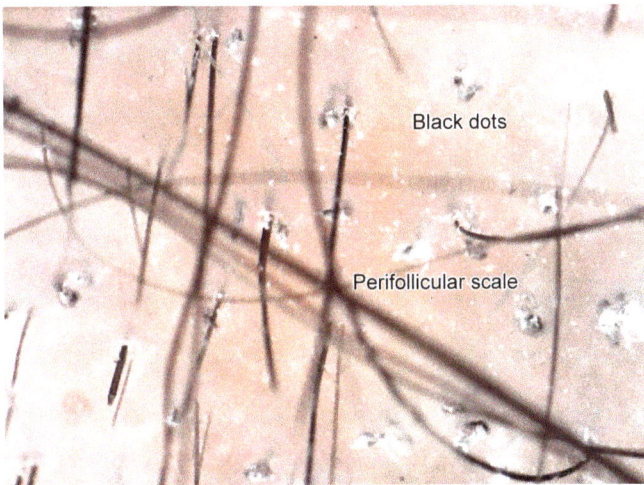

Fig. 5: Dermatoscopic image showing extensive perifollicular scaling along with black dots.

SECTION 3: Diagnosis of Dermatophytosis

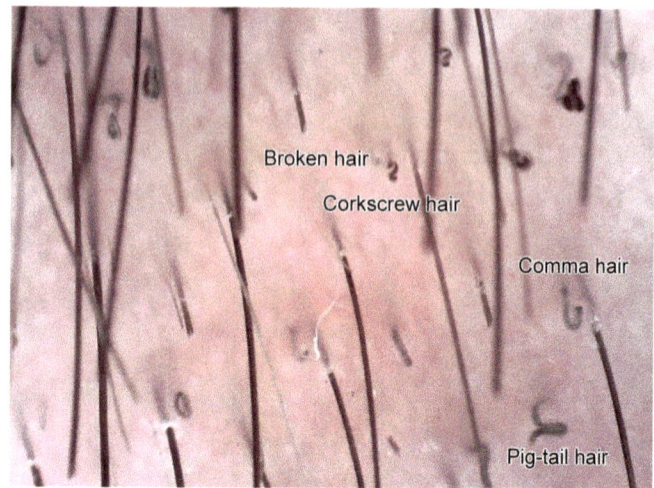

Fig. 6: Dermatoscopic image showing curved hair of various morphologies.

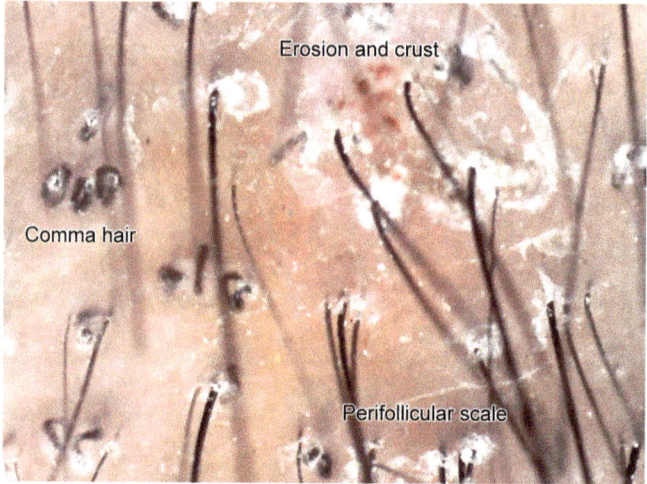

Fig. 7: Dermatoscopic image showing inflammatory changes with erosions and crusts along with other changes of tinea infection.

Tinea of Glabrous Skin

Dermatophyte skin infection is the least studied entity of the three. Not many studies are available. However, in the setting of altered tinea presentations, it assumes a greater diagnostic significance in view of

CHAPTER 11: Dermatoscopy (Skin, Hair, and Nail) and Bedside Diagnosis...

TABLE 2: Dermoscopic findings in tinea capitis.	
Dermoscopic findings	**Features**
Characteristic findings with a high predictive value but not seen in every case	Comma hairs (short hairs that bend and grow back toward the scalp, resembling a comma)
	Corkscrew hairs (short hairs that are coiled up like a corkscrew). Typical of *Trichophyton* infection and are seen less commonly in infection due to *Microsporum canis*
	Zigzag hairs (short hairs with several bends in them like a zigzag pattern)
	Barcode-like (Morse code-like) hairs
	Bent hairs
Common dermoscopic findings, but which are not diagnostic	Scale, follicular keratosis, and crusts
	Erythema
	Broken hairs and black dots

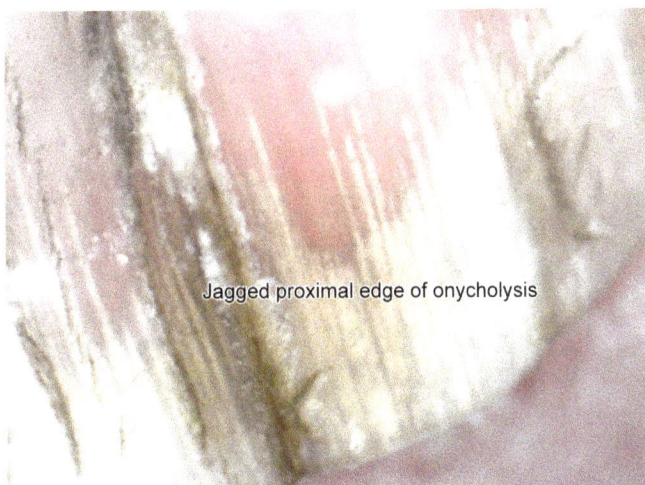

Fig. 8: Dermatoscopic image showing proximal jagged edge of onycholysis in tinea unguium.

the subtle clues it offers toward suggesting tinea infection as well as suggesting topical steroid abuse. The background nonspecific erythema is seen in most steroid-modified tinea lesions. There can be presence of micropustules as well as broad telangiectasia (which suggests steroid abuse). The lesional scale is mostly marginal, when present. Even though

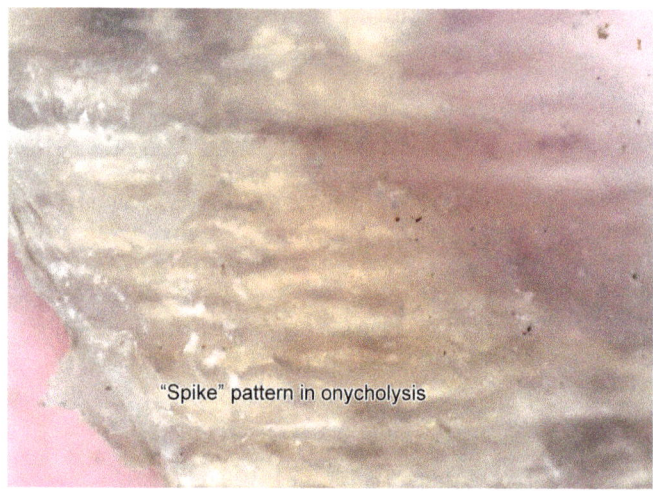

Fig. 9: Dermatoscopic image showing the presence of spikes within the onycholyzed area.

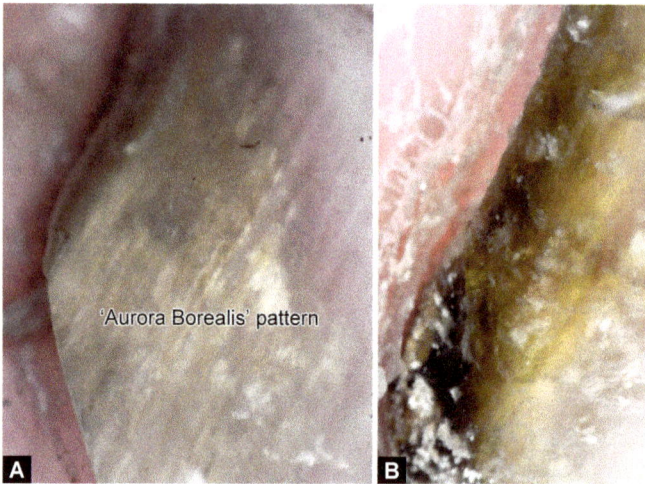

Figs. 10A and B: Dermatoscopic image showing spectrum of color changes through the nail plate, the so-called Aurora Borealis pattern.

CHAPTER 11: Dermatoscopy (Skin, Hair, and Nail) and Bedside Diagnosis...

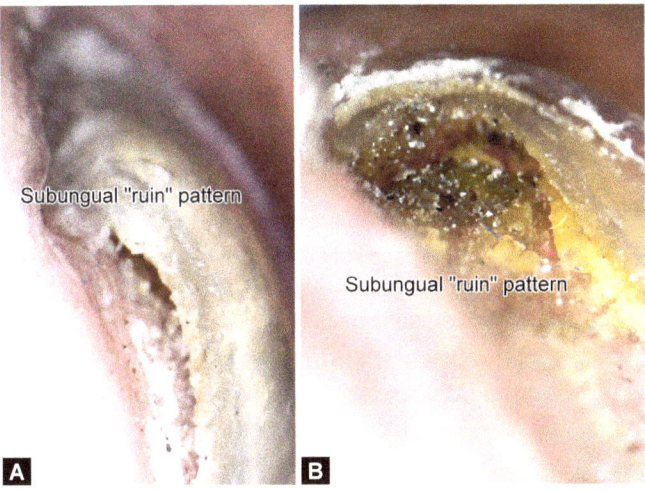

Figs. 11A and B: Dermatoscopic image of the distal edge showing subungual ruin appearance.

TABLE 3: Dermoscopic findings in onychomycosis.	
Type of onychomycosis	**Onychoscopy features**
Distal lateral subungual onychomycosis	• Jagged edge of onycholysis with spikes (whitish longitudinal lines) on the proximal end of the onycholytic area • "Aurora Borealis" pattern—longitudinal striae of varying colors, white/yellow/brown/occasionally green within the onycholytic nail plate • Subungual "ruinous" appearance of the subungual hyperkeratosis • Distal irregular termination—distal pulverization of the thickened nail plate • Fungal melanonychia-multicolored pigmentation: Yellow/brown/gray/black/red which is wider in the distal end (black reverse triangle) in association with thick subungual hyperkeratosis • Leukonychia—homogenous/punctate • Superficial transverse striation—fine onychoschizia
Dermatophytoma	Round yellow–orange subungual area, connected by a thin band to the distal edge of the nail plate

Continued

Continued

Type of onychomycosis	Onychoscopy features
Superficial white onychomycosis	• White, opaque, friable spots of scaling distributed irregularly along the nail • As compared to keratin granulation where firmly attached scales are seen only distally • Application of interface media leads to disappearance of scales • Grid pattern of scaling
Endonyx onychomycosis	• Onychoschizia • Absence of subungual hyperkeratosis or onycholysis • Milky white leukonychia • Dendritic pattern
Proximal subungual onychomycosis	• White discoloration below the nail plate in the lunula • White patches with advancing linear distal edges

it may not be visible to naked eye, it is relatively easier to visualize on dermoscopy. The scale can also be perifollicular or localized to creases.

The involvement of body hair or vellus hair visible on dermoscopy is of particular diagnostic and prognostic value. It predicts possibility of poor response to therapy and need for prolonged oral therapy even if it is localized tinea. Invasion of hair follicles and short nonpigmented vellus hair is common in steroid-modified cases.

Nowadays, it is very pertinent to be able to diagnose atypical lesions of tinea. Diagnosis is mostly based on clinical clues. However, dermatoscopy offers pertinent clues in this scenario as it shows characteristic fungal hair involvement in the form of broken hair, translucent hair, bent hair, or coiled hair. The background erythema along with extensive steroid induced telangiectasia can help offer clues toward the cause of recalcitrance. Presence of pustules which may not be apparent to the naked eye is also a valuable clue. Other than this, dermoscopy can help delineate the fine marginal scaling in cases with tinea incognito where clinically apparent marginal scale is not discernible.

Dermoscopic findings in tinea corporis, cruris, etc., are summarized in **Table 4** and depicted in **Figures 12 to 16**.

TABLE 4: Dermoscopic findings in dermatophytic skin infections.

Type of cutaneous fungal infection	Dermoscopic features
Tinea corporis	• Diffuse erythema • Whitish scales, especially peripherally • Follicular micropustules, especially peripherally • Brown spots surrounded by a white-yellowish halo • Wavy hair, broken hair within the lesion • Morse code hairs of vellus hairs
Tinea cruris	• Features similar to tinea corporis • Morse code hair • Easily deformable hair • Transparent hair
Tinea manuum or pedis	• Whitish scales along the palmar and plantar creases • Brownish scales showing dried vesicles • Areas of intense erythema
Tinea incognito	• Morse code hairs • Damaged vellus hairs • Follicular micropustules • Concentric areas of erythema separated by scales • Easily deformable hairs that look transparent • Bent hair • Telangiectasia

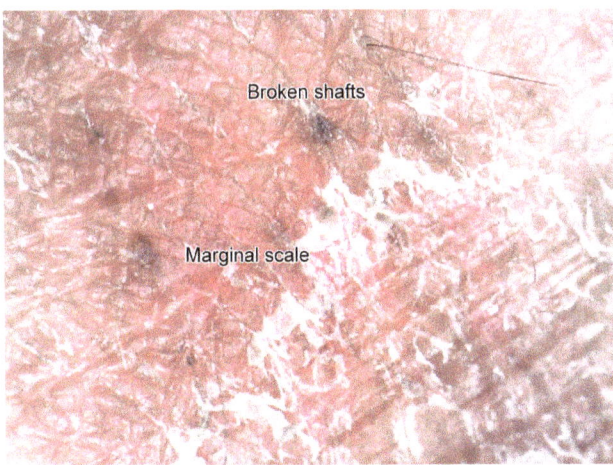

Fig. 12: Dermatoscopic image showing marginal scale of tinea which was hardly visible on naked eye examination. Broken hair shafts as suggested by black dots, show extensive follicle involvement.

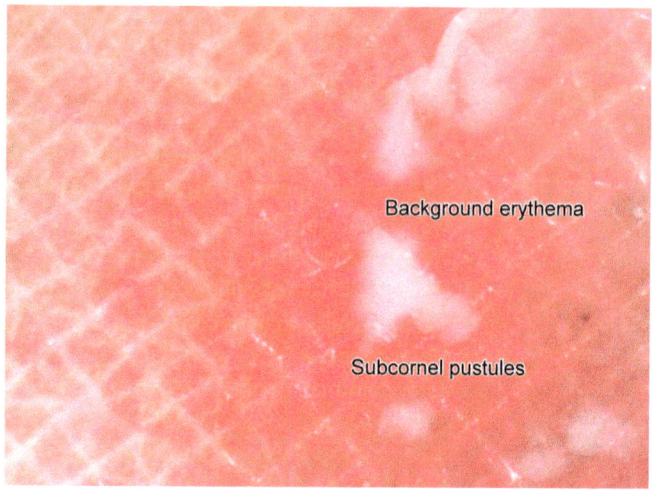

Fig. 13: Dermatoscopic image showing extensive background erythema with superficial pustules in a steroid-modified tinea.

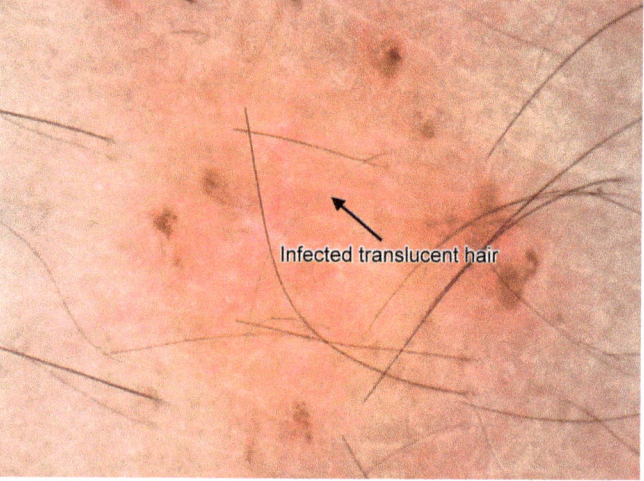

Fig. 14: Dermatoscopic image showing an infected translucent hair.

CHAPTER 11: Dermatoscopy (Skin, Hair, and Nail) and Bedside Diagnosis...

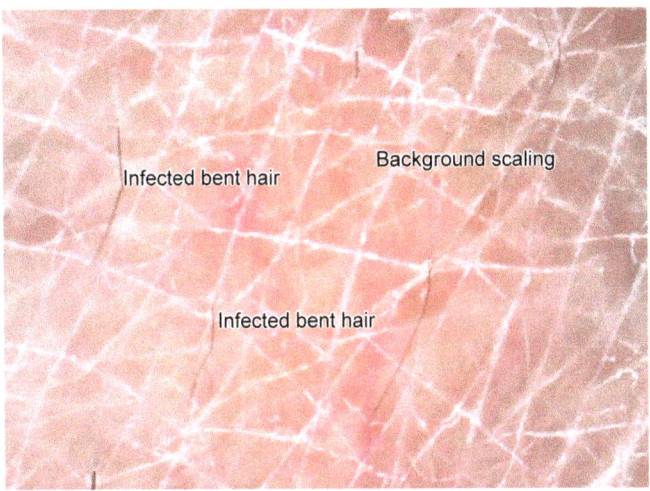

Fig. 15: Dermatoscopic image showing multiple bent hair, possibly infected, with background scaling accentuated in skin creases.

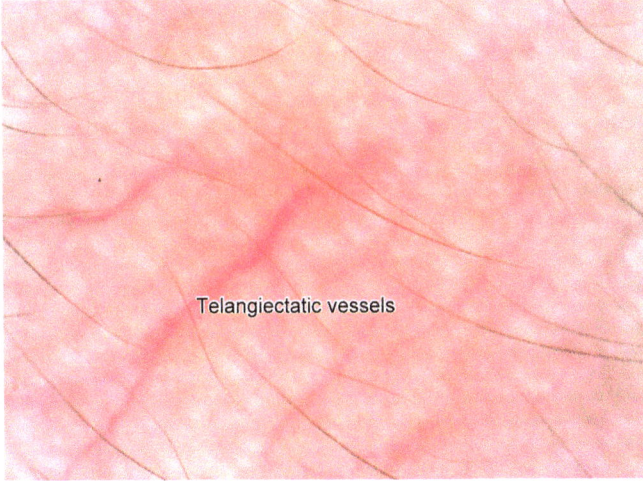

Fig. 16: Dermatoscopic image showing broad telangiectatic vessels due to prolonged steroid abuse.

CHAPTER 12

Laboratory Diagnosis

DIRECT MICROSCOPIC EXAMINATION

Direct examination under the microscope is the simplest and quickest method to diagnose superficial fungal infections. A thin layer of sample collected is mounted on a glass slide with potassium hydroxide (KOH 10-30%). The KOH causes destruction of keratin squames without affecting the fungus. Gentle heating of the slide accelerates the process, which might be needed in nail specimens. The skin and hair samples can be seen under the microscope immediately, while nail samples usually take few hours for preparation. The nail samples can be kept overnight before reporting it as negative. The alternative is addition of 35% dimethyl sulfoxide (DMSO), dimethylacetamide, or dimethyl formamide to KOH to hasten the process of softening. Apart from this, some stains like Congo red, methylene blue, cotton blue, and Parker's blue ink can be used to increase the contrast between the hyphae and the debris. Fluorescent microscopes, if available, can be helpful by staining the samples with calcofluor-white (CFW) or acridine orange. The sensitivity of this test is high for cutaneous infections but varies from approximately 50-85% for cases with onychomycosis.

FUNGAL CULTURE

Fungal culture is essential in cases where long-term systemic antifungal therapy is required, for example, onychomycosis and tinea capitis. A positive test takes around 7-21 days depending upon the causative fungus. The most common primary culture medium used is Sabouraud's dextrose agar (SDA) which is composed of 4% sugar, 1% peptone, and has an acidic pH. An antibacterial agent, like chloramphenicol (0.005%) or gentamicin (0.0025%), is usually added to avoid bacterial contamination of the growth. Additionally, to ensure isolation of dermatophytes, cycloheximide (0.04%) is also added to inhibit nondermatophytic mold (NDM) growth **(Figs. 1 to 3)**.

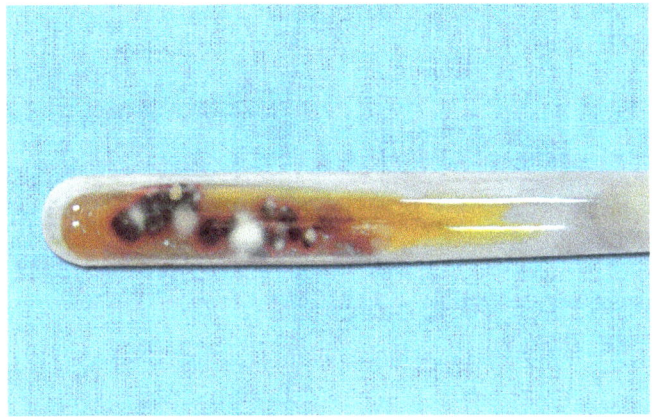

Fig. 1: Positive culture for fungi on medium—SDA or chrome agar in tubes.
(SDA: Sabouraud's dextrose agar)

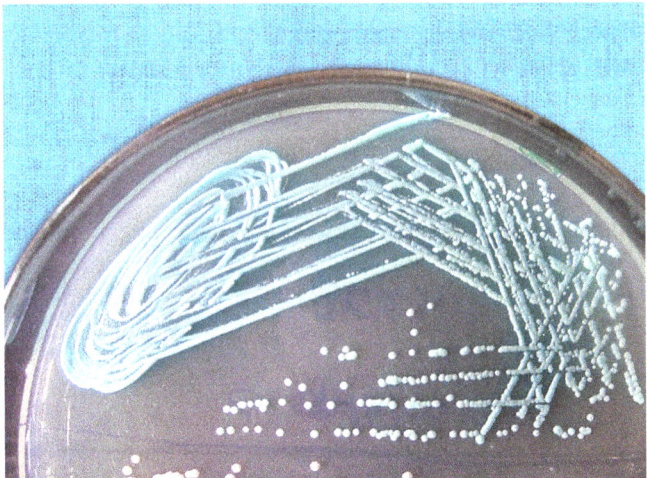

Fig. 2: Positive culture for fungi on SDA medium in a plate.
(SDA: Sabouraud's dextrose agar)

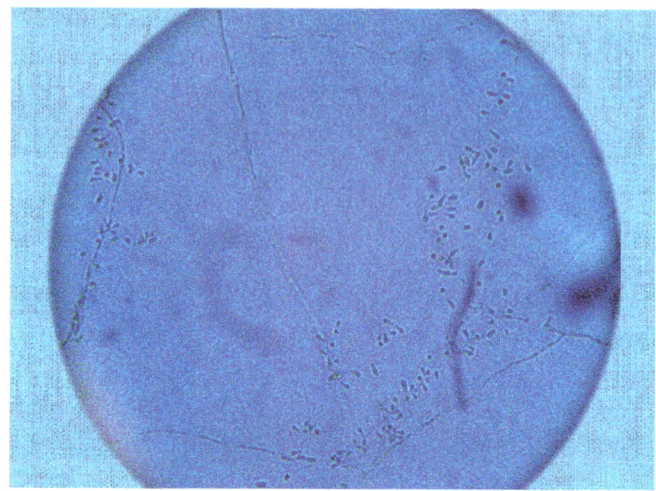

Fig. 3: Subsequently, lactophenol cotton blue mounts are prepared for species identification.

HISTOPATHOLOGY

Histopathology is generally not required for diagnosis of superficial fungal infections However, in diagnostic challenge cases, especially those involving nail, histopathology with special stains for fungus can help document actual fungal invasion. It may also be required in cases with extensive steroid-modified tinea, or tinea erythroderma, where other diagnoses need to be ruled out.

INVESTIGATIONS

The diagnosis of a suspected dermatophytic infection is confirmed by direct microscopy followed by fungal culture. Fungal culture is not done routinely for all cases, except for those with onychomycosis or tinea capitis, in which long duration of treatment is warranted.

Direct Microscopy

On direct microscopic examination, the dermatophytes can be seen as septate hyphae with an even diameter along their length. In case of hair invasion, four distinct patterns can be visualized as enumerated above **(Fig. 4)**.

CHAPTER 12: Laboratory Diagnosis   93

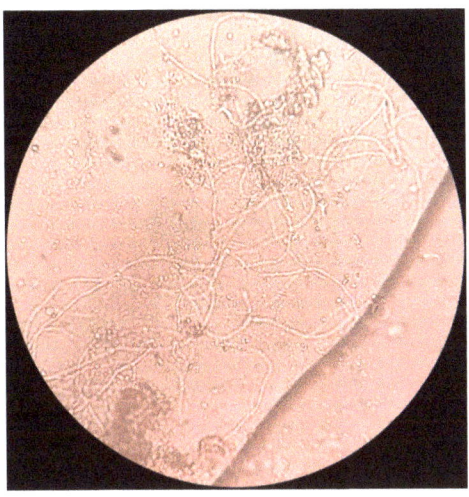

Fig. 4: Presence of dermatophyte septate hyphae under low power [potassium hydroxide (KOH) mount 400×].

Fungal Culture

Culture is usually done in SDA (with chloramphenicol and cycloheximide) at 26–28°C, in which the dermatophytes grow readily. Cultures should be incubated for 3 weeks before reporting it as negative.

Histopathology

Histopathology is a useful investigation in cases of nail invasion, especially when repeated direct microcopy and cultures are negative. It can help in ruling out other close differential diagnoses. In histopathological specimens, hyphae can be seen with periodic acid–Schiff (PAS) stain inside the lamellar structure of the nail plate, lying parallel to its surface **(Fig. 5)**. The epidermis may show spongiosis with focal parakeratosis. Other stains like Grocott methenamine silver (GMS) and CFW can also be used to increase the sensitivity. Histopathology cannot identify the species or differentiate between viable and nonviable organisms.

The difficulty in diagnosing fungal nail invasion has spurred interest in evaluating newer diagnostic options, especially useful for onychomycosis. These include polymerase chain reaction (PCR) techniques, optical coherence tomography, confocal laser scan microscopy, and phase contrast hard X-ray microscopy. MALDI-TOF (matrix-assisted laser

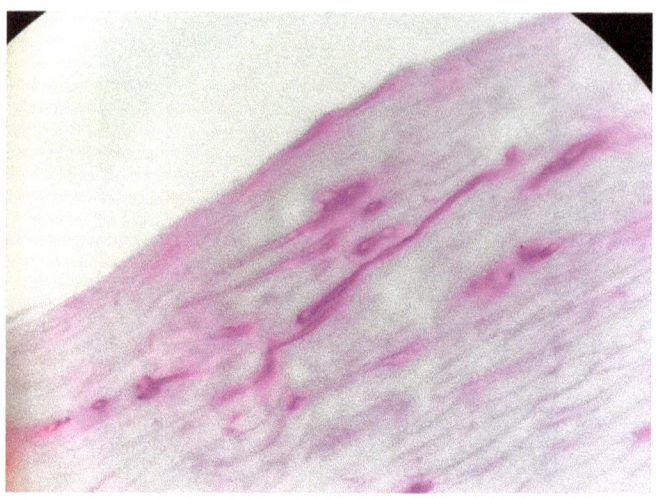

Fig. 5: Fungal invasion in the nail plate structure [periodic acid–Schiff (PAS) stained nail plate biopsy 400×].

desorption ionization-time of flight) mass spectrometry is perceived as a promising experimental technique but not as a practical tool in the real world.

DIAGNOSIS

The confirmation of diagnosis of candidiasis is simply by demonstration of typical budding yeast cells (2-6 × 3-9 μm) **(Fig. 6)** with a narrow base accompanied by hyphae or pseudohyphae (except for *Candida glabrata*) by light microscopy. *Candida albicans* grows easily on cycloheximide free SDA at 37°C; whitish mucoid colonies appear in 2-5 days. However, the plate should be incubated for 1 week before reporting it as negative. CHROMagar *Candida* is a new medium that is used for isolation and identification of some clinically important species and can differentiate between different species on the basis of color produced by the fungal colonies. It is important to identify the species implicated, as some nonalbicans species like *C. glabrata* and *Candida krusei* show primary fluconazole resistance. The characteristic feature of *C. albicans* is the ability to produce germ tubes when incubated in serum at 37°C for 2-4 hours. The only other species that can produce germ tube is *Candida dubliniensis*, known to cause oral thrush in HIV-positive patients.

CHAPTER 12: Laboratory Diagnosis

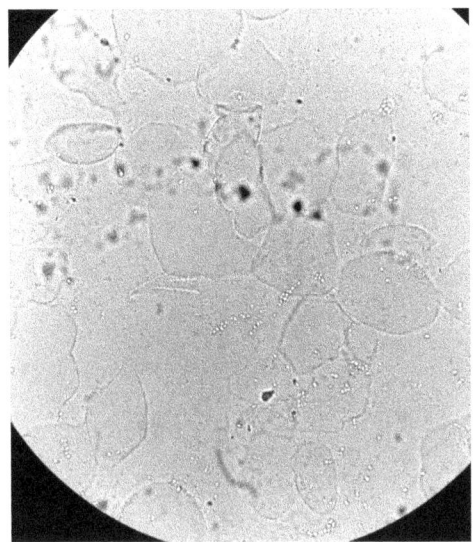

Fig. 6: *Candida* pseudohyphae and budding yeasts [potassium hydroxide (KOH) mount 400×].

Histopathology from the satellite pustule shows subcorneal neutrophil accumulation. The yeast cells can be demonstrated in stratum corneum with PAS stain or methenamine silver stain. In disseminated candidiasis, an organism is seen inside the blood vessels by special stains.

SECTION 4

Treatment of Dermatophytosis

Chapter 13: General Measures
Chapter 14: Topical Therapy
Chapter 15: Systemic Treatment
Chapter 16: Systemic Treatment in Special Populations

CHAPTER 13

General Measures

INTRODUCTION

It is a challenging job for the physician to treat the so-called innocuous dermatophytic infections. General measures are extremely important to improve the treatment outcome, reducing the duration of therapy, preventing the spread to close contacts as well as preventing the recurrences in these days of recalcitrant dermatophytosis.

The important general measures have been summarized in **Box 1**.

BOX 1 | **General measures to be followed by patients of dermatophytoses.**

- Daily bath and adequate drying of the skin with special attention to flexural areas such as axillae, groins, interdigital web spaces, and infra- and intermammary folds in females
- Avoid using tight occlusive or body-hugging clothing such as jeans/synthetic clothing
- Use of loose cotton clothing in summers
- Regular washing of personal clothes, towels, and bed linen and drying them in sun as sunlight is known to kill dermatophytes
- If there is no sun, patients should be advised to iron clothes including undergarments
- No sharing of towels or clothing with siblings/friends
- Wash infected clothing separately
- Avoidance of body-contact sports and swimming is preferable
- Simultaneous treatment of affected family members is vital to prevent reinfection
- Stressing on the importance of regularity of medication and adherence to the treatment duration for both topical and systemic antifungal treatment
- The topical antifungals should be applied 2 cm beyond the margin of the lesion for at least 2 weeks beyond the clinical resolution of skin lesions. We call this recommendation of applying topical antifungals 2 cm beyond the margin, twice a day for 2 weeks beyond clinical resolution "The rule of two"

CHAPTER 14

Topical Therapy

INTRODUCTION

Topical antifungals are various creams, solutions, lotions, powders, gels, sprays, or lacquers, which can be applied on mucocutaneous surface to treat a fungal infection. Many topical antifungal medications are suitable for both dermatophyte and yeast infections; while some maybe specific to one or the other type of fungus. Topical antifungals were conventionally considered useful for treating tinea infections other than tinea capitis and tinea unguium. However, with the advent of recalcitrant dermatophytoses, their use has become limited. At the same time, they have an important role to play in some cases of onychomycosis, for long-term maintenance, and prevention of relapse in treated cases. Many of these agents have a broad spectrum of activity, being effective against dermatophytes, yeasts, and *Malassezia furfur*.

Topical antifungals are broadly of two types: specific and nonspecific agents. The specific antifungals include the polyenes, azoles, allylamines, amorolfine, ciclopirox, and butenafine. The nonspecific agents include Whitfield's ointment or keratolytics for limited use. Most topical antifungals act on the fungal cell wall formation, by inhibiting the production of an important component ergosterol.

Topical antifungal drugs can also be classified based on their chemical structure which also determines their mechanism of action. The four categories are summarized in **Table 1**.

Although, similar antifungal agents (topical or systemic) are used for the treatment of most of these infections, the treatment regimens vary according to the site being treated. The commonly used topical antifungals are summarized in **Table 2**.

CHAPTER 14: Topical Therapy

TABLE 1: Different types of topical antifungals and their mechanisms of action.

Category	Examples	Mechanism of action
Azoles	• *Imidazoles*: Clotrimazole, Econazole, Ketoconazole, Miconazole, Tioconazole, Efinaconazole, etc. • *Triazoles*: Fluconazole	• Target ergosterol biosynthesis by inhibiting C-14 α-demethylase • Prevent demethylation of lanosterol to ergosterol, inciting a cascade of membrane defects • Predominantly fungistatic
Polyenes	Nystatin	• Binds to ergosterol in fungal cell membrane • Promote leakage of intracellular ions, disrupt active transport mechanisms • Can be fungistatic or fungicidal
Allylamines	Naftifine, terbinafine	• Competitive inhibition of squalene epoxidase, blocking conversion of squalene to lanosterol • Resultant squalene accumulation and ergosterol depletion in cell membrane • Fungicidal in action
Benzoxaboroles	Tavaborole	• Inhibits leucyl-tRNA synthetase (LeuRS) via the oxaborole tRNA trapping mechanism • Anti-inflammatory and antimicrobial activities (including antifungal, antimalarial, antitrypanosomal, ectoparasiticide, anticancer, antipneumococcal and antitubercular)
Others	Amorolfine (morpholine derivative), ciclopirox, thiocarbamate antifungals, undecylenic alkanolamide antifungals, tolnaftate	Varied

TABLE 2: Commonly used topical antifungal drugs, their formulations, and expected adverse effects.

Drug	Formulations	Mechanism of action	Common reported side effects
Azoles: • Clotrimazole • Miconazole • Econazole • Sertaconazole • Luliconazole • Oxiconazole • Eberconazole	Cream, lotion, powder	Inhibition of ergosterol synthesis	Rare, itching, burning
Azoles: Efinaconazole	Nail solution	Inhibition of ergosterol synthesis	Rare, itching, burning
Allylamines (terbinafine)	Cream	Inhibition of squalene epoxidase	Rare, itching, burning, rash
Tolnaftate	Cream	Inhibition of squalene epoxidase	Skin irritation—redness, burning
• Ciclopirox olamine • Piroctone olamine	Cream, shampoo, nail lacquer	Chelates polyvalent metal cations, such as Fe^{3+} and Al^{3+}	Skin irritation
Amorolfine	Cream, nail lacquer	Inhibits ergosterol synthesis at two steps: The delta 14 reduction and the delta 7–8 isomerization	Redness, itching
Benzoxaboroles: Tavaborole	Nail solution	Inhibition of leucyl-tRNA synthetase (LeuRS)	Rare, itching, burning

Topical nail lacquers such as ciclopirox 8% and amorolfine 5% can be used alone or in combination with systemic antifungals. The common side effects of nail lacquer include transient periungual erythema or burning at the site of application; and bluish or yellowish-brown discoloration with the use of amorolfine, which clears upon discontinuing treatment.

USE OF TOPICAL ANTIFUNGALS IN SUPERFICIAL DERMATOPHYTOSIS

Prior to using topical antifungals, wash the affected area with soap and water and dry it completely. Wash both hands thoroughly after applying topical preparations. Apply a thin layer of topical antifungals to the area of infection. Avoid using occlusion or wrapping. Patients are advised to apply 2 cm beyond the margin of the lesions. The use and choice of topical antifungals is determined by the type of dermatophytosis, described in the following text.

Tinea Capitis

Systemic antifungals remain the mainstay of therapy as topical drugs cannot achieve effective penetration into the hair shaft. Antifungal shampoos containing ketoconazole or selenium sulfide have been found to reduce spore shedding and hence, prevent transmission to close contacts. Ciclopirox olamine or piroctone olamine containing lotions can also be use, though they are more useful in patients with seborrheic dermatitis. Scalp hygiene and avoiding sharing of combs and pillow cases are other measures advised to reduce the potential of transmission.

Tinea Corporis/Cruris/Faciei

For localized disease, topical antifungals such as miconazole, clotrimazole, terbinafine, and tolnaftate are usually sufficient. The drug needs to be applied twice daily for approximately 4 weeks. For extensive skin areas, systemic treatment is usually recommended.

Tinea Barbae

Tinea barbae, being an extensive hair infection, needs to be treated with oral antifungals, just as tinea capitis.

Tinea Pedis and Manuum

Cases with mild interdigital involvement can usually be treated with topical azoles, allylamines, or tolnaftate. However, for almost all infections including chronic hyperkeratotic type of infection, oral antifungals are essential for cure. Topical antifungals can aid an early response as well as prevention of relapse.

Tinea Unguium

Due to the limited drug penetration as well as slow rate of nail growth, tinea unguium requires long-term treatment with oral antifungals. The choice of treatment depends on the type of nail invasion and the species involved. Topical treatment options are also available with enhanced drug delivery systems, but are usually recommended in cases without any matrix involvement; involvement of <50% of distal nail plate; or those with contraindications to oral antifungals. Topical and systemic therapies can also be combined to hasten the cure and ensure broader spectrum coverage.

Topical antifungals found useful in nail are the two recently the Food and Drug Administration (FDA)-approved drugs (Efinaconazole and Tavaborole—both as solutions) and the older nail lacquers (ciclopirox and amorolfine). The nail surface has to be cleaned before application, and the drugs have to be used as per their specified schedule. Daily application and a long duration of treatment (up to 48 weeks) are required. Ciclopirox and amorolfine lacquers penetrate through nail but have low efficacy as monotherapy. Tavaborole and efinaconazole have to be applied under the nail.

- *Ciclopirox*, a fungicidal drug, interferes with the synthesis of DNA, RNA, and protein by inhibiting the transport of essential elements in fungal cells. It has broad-spectrum activity against dermatophytes, yeast and nondermatophyte molds (NDM) such as *Scopulariopsis brevicaulis, Aspergillus niger, A. fumigatus,* and *Scytalidium dimidiatum*. It is to be used once daily on affected nail(s) for up to 48 weeks producing mycological cure rates of 47–67%, and complete cure rate of 25%. Adverse effects include transient irritation, burning, or itching.
- *Amorolfine* (morpholine derivative) is also broad-spectrum fungicidal and fungistatic. The lacquer is to be applied once or twice per week for 24–48 weeks, producing clinical cure ranging from 38 to 54%. Adverse effects are uncommon and mild including local irritation, onycholysis, and contact dermatitis and nail discoloration.
- *Efinaconazole* is approved for onychomycosis of the toenail(s) due to *Trichophyton rubrum* and *T. mentagrophytes*. It produces complete cure in 17.8–15.2% patients and mycologic cure in 53.4–55.2% at 48 weeks. Efinaconazole is a topical triazole which is fungistatic. It is available as a 10% solution.

- *Tavaborole* is also indicated for toenail onychomycosis due to *Trichophyton rubrum* or *Trichophyton mentagrophytes*. At 48 weeks, it produced complete cure in 6.5–9.1% patients while mycological cure in 31.1–35.9%. Tavaborole is available as 5% topical solution.

Two other topicals with limited efficacy data in onychomycosis include terbinafine nail lacquer (not widely studied, though it has shown efficacy superior to ciclopirox) and Luliconazole 5% solution (which has been approved for once daily application in onychomycosis).

ADVERSE EFFECTS

Topical antifungal medications usually come with side effects. These include itching, and local irritations with few products. Rarely, signs of increased irritation or possible sensitization may be seen. These include pruritus, burning sensation, oozing, and vesiculation. Topical antifungal drugs may also interact with food and different medications. Therefore, they should be used with caution and with proper advice and expectations.

DEVICE-BASED THERAPIES

Low cure rates and high relapse rates in dermatophytosis, especially onychomycosis, are seen even with highly efficacious antifungals. This has led to the development of newer treatment options to ensure drug penetration, drug persistence, mycological cure, and effective prevention of relapse. These include device-related therapies and physical measures to enhance drug penetration through nail, and development of synergistic combinations. There are the Food and Drug Administration (FDA)-approved laser systems: PinPointe (NuvoLase Inc, Chico, CA, USA) and Genesis Plus (Cutera Inc, CA, USA), both approved to produce a temporary enhancement of clear nail in patients with onychomycosis. Potential phototherapy treatments for onychomycosis have been evaluated in podiatric literature. These include light-based technologies including ultraviolet light therapy, near infrared photo inactivation therapy, and photothermal ablative antisepsis, for use in onychomycosis. Surgical avulsion followed by topical therapies can be considered for single nail onychomycosis, not responsive to standard therapies or infection with nondermatophyte species; however, the results are not very encouraging.

CHAPTER 15

Systemic Treatment

INTRODUCTION

The therapeutic armamentarium for the antifungal drugs used in the management of superficial dermatophytosis is very small. Commonly used antifungal drugs have been listed in **Table 1** with their mechanism of action and side effect profile.

Table 2 illustrates dosing schedules for dermatophytosis involving different body parts.

Terbinafine, a squalene epoxide inhibitor, is a fungicidal drug. It is well absorbed orally and is recommended in a dose of 250 mg once a day for 6 weeks and 12 weeks for finger and toe nails, respectively. Common adverse reactions include gastrointestinal symptoms, skin rash, pruritus, urticaria, asymptomatic liver enzyme abnormalities and taste disturbances.

TABLE 1: Common systemic antifungal drugs.

Drug	Antifungal effect	Mechanism of action	Common reported side effects
Griseofulvin (micronized formulation)	Fungistatic	Inhibition of intracellular microtubules	Headache, nausea, exacerbation of SLE, porphyria
Ketoconazole, fluconazole and itraconazole	Fungistatic	Inhibition of ergosterol synthesis	Hepatitis (most common with ketoconazole), headache, nausea
Terbinafine	Fungicidal	Inhibition of squalene epoxidase	Gastrointestinal disturbance, skin rash, pruritus, taste disturbance, rarely hepatitis

(SLE: systemic lupus erythematosus)

TABLE 2: Treatment regimen for common dermatophytoses.

Indication	Drug	Dosage	Minimum duration of therapy (May need to be prolonged depending on the basis of resistant and recalcitrant infection)
Tinea unguium (onychomycosis)	Terbinafine	250 mg OD	6 weeks for finger nails, 12 weeks for toe nails

	Itraconazole	200 mg BD	• 1 week for each month for:
			  ○ Consecutive 2 months for fingernails
			  ○ Consecutive 3 months for toe nails

	Fluconazole	150–300 mg/week	Around 9–12 months
Tinea corporis/ cruris/faciei	Terbinafine	250 mg OD	2–4 weeks
	Itraconazole	100 mg OD	1–2 weeks
	Fluconazole	150 mg/week	2–4 weeks
Tinea capitis	Griseofulvin	5–25 mg/kg/day	6–8 weeks
	Terbinafine	250 mg/day (adults > 40kg) • 125 mg/day (20–40 kg) • 62.5 mg/day (<20 kg)	4–6 weeks
Tinea pedis/ manuum	Terbinafine	250 mg OD	2 weeks
	Itraconazole	200 mg BD	7 days
Tinea barbae	Griseofulvin	1 g OD	4–6 weeks
	Terbinafine	250 mg OD	

Itraconazole, a triazole antifungal, has broadest antifungal spectrum. It can be used either in continuous form or as pulse therapy. In pulse form, itraconazole 200 mg twice a day is recommended for 7 days a month. The usual time period of therapy is 2-3 cycles in finger nails and 3-4 cycles in toenails. In continuous therapy, itraconazole is given daily in the dose of 200 mg for 3 months. This regimen is more expensive as well as more prone to side effects as compared to the pulse regimen.

Fluconazole is not recommended as first-line therapy for tinea unguium, because of its prolonged treatment period and lack of supportive efficacy data. The cure rate is expectedly lower as compared to terbinafine and itraconazole. The usual recommended dose is 150-300 mg weekly. The common reported adverse effects include gastrointestinal upset, headache and skin rash.

Griseofulvin is now replaced by newer antifungals. It has the lowest cure rate and requires long-term treatment (6-12 months). So, it is not usually recommended for the treatment of tinea unguium.

TINEA CAPITIS

Systemic antifungals remain the mainstay of therapy as topical drugs cannot achieve effective penetration into the hair shaft. The most common oral antifungal used is griseofulvin which remains the standard therapy for tinea capitis because of its long-standing safety and efficacy profile in children. The conventional dose depends on the formulation being used. For the ultra-micronized form, it is 10 mg/kg/day and for the micronized form, it is 20 mg/kg/day, given for a period of 6-8 weeks. Griseofulvin works better on *Microsporum* species. The reported side effects include headache, photosensitivity, and gastrointestinal side effects. Fluconazole in the dose of 5 mg/kg/day for 4-6 weeks is effective against *Trichophyton* species. It is reported to be much safer as compared to ketoconazole in terms of hepatic profile. Itraconazole (3-5 mg/kg/ day) for 4-6 weeks is reported to be effective. The side effects include diarrhea, gastrointestinal upset and rarely, hepatitis and congestive heart failure. Terbinafine (3-6 mg/kg/day or 62.5-250 mg/day) is found to more effective against *Trichophyton violaceum* and *Trichophyton tonsurans* species and usually therapy is needed for 2-4 weeks.

Antifungal shampoos containing ketoconazole or selenium sulfide have been found to reduce spore shedding and hence, prevent transmission to close contacts. Scalp hygiene and avoiding sharing of combs and pillow cases are other measures advised to reduce the potential of transmission.

TINEA CORPORIS/CRURIS/FACIEI

For localized disease, topical antifungals such as miconazole, clotrimazole, terbinafine, and tolnaftate are usually sufficient. The drug needs to be applied twice daily for approximately 2-4 weeks. For extensive skin areas, systemic treatment with terbinafine or itraconazole in standard doses is usually recommended. Oral griseofulvin and fluconazole are also effective but require longer treatment period.

TINEA BARBAE

Tinea barbae, being an extensive hair infection, needs to be treated with oral antifungals, just as tinea capitis. The usual time period for continuation of therapy is 4-6 weeks.

TINEA PEDIS AND TINEA MANUUM

Cases with mild interdigital involvement can usually be treated with topical azoles, allylamines, or tolnaftate. However, for almost all infections including chronic hyperkeratotic type of infection, oral antifungals like terbinafine, fluconazole, or itraconazole are essential for producing a cure.

TINEA UNGUIUM

Due to the limited drug penetration as well as slow rate of nail growth, tinea unguium requires long-term treatment with oral antifungals. The choice of treatment depends on the type of nail invasion and the species involved. Topical treatment options are also available with enhanced drug delivery systems, but are usually recommended in cases without any matrix involvement; involvement of <50% of distal nail plate; or those with contraindications to oral antifungals. Topical and systemic therapies can also be combined to hasten the cure and ensure broader spectrum coverage.

TRICHOPHYTON RUBRUM SYNDROME

This is a particularly extensive and recalcitrant form of tinea infection. The treatment recommendations are summarized in **Box 1**.

SECTION 4: Treatment of Dermatophytosis

> **BOX 1** **Management recommendations for *Trichophyton rubrum* syndrome.**
>
> - Identify predisposing host environmental factors
> - Establish the diagnosis (diagnostic criteria detailed before)
> - Check for causes of immunosuppression (such as HIV infection, immunosuppressive drug intake), which may suggest an alternative diagnosis
> - Antifungals:
>   - To be used for prolonged periods—can go up to 3 months
>   - They may have to be combined with other antifungals, some options include:
>   - Itraconazole 200 mg/day for 4–6 weeks (may extend till complete resolution)
>   - Combination of itraconazole 200 mg/day and terbinafine 250 mg/day for 4–6 weeks or extended periods
>   - Itraconazole 200 mg twice a day for 7 days every month for 3–5 months depending on clinical response
>   - Topical luliconazole/sertaconazole for up to 6 weeks
>   - Topical terbinafine/amorolfine/ciclopirox twice daily for extended periods
> - Taking care of fomites and household contact
> - Assuring patient compliance till complete clearance

CHAPTER 16

Systemic Treatment in Special Populations

INTRODUCTION

Treatment of dermatophytosis in special population groups such as pregnant and lactating women, extremes of ages (children and elderly) and patient with liver and renal disease needs a cautious approach and special considerations. In pregnancy and lactation, all oral agents are best avoided and topical antifungal treatment is preferred. Same goes for very young and very old patients. Elderly people are of special concerns as they are likely to have age related comorbidities and are on polypharmacy. Therefore, extreme care should be exercised while prescribing oral antifungal to avoid drug-related side effects resulting from drug interactions. Though ample evidence of safety of terbinafine and itraconazole exists in children and elderly, terbinafine is preferred drug.

Table 1 details the safety profile of different oral antifungals that are used for dermatophytosis in special population.

TABLE 1: Safety profile of oral antifungals in special population.

Drug	Pregnancy and lactation	Elderly	Liver disease	Renal disease
Griseofulvin	Not recommended	May be given	C/I	May be given
Terbinafine	• Not recommended • Category B may be given in 2nd and 3rd trimesters with great caution	May be prescribed with regular monitoring	C/I	Use with caution with regular laboratory monitoring

Continued

Continued

Drug	Pregnancy and lactation	Elderly	Liver disease	Renal disease
Itraconazole	• Category-C • Not recommended	Use with caution C/I with cardiac disease	May be given	C/I
Fluconazole	• Category-C • Not recommended	Use with caution with regular LFT monitoring	C/I	Dose adjustment needed

(C/I: contraindicated; LFT: liver function test)

Advisory on the dosing schedule of different antifungals for children has been detailed in **Table 2**.

TABLE 2: Weight-wise dosage of systemic antifungal for children.			
Weight	Terbinafine	Itraconazole	Fluconazole
<20 kg	62.5 mg/day	5 mg/kg/day	3–6 mg/kg/day
20–40 kg	125 mg/day	100 mg/day	3–6 mg/kg/day
>40 kg	250 mg/day	200 mg/day	3–6 mg/kg/day

SECTION 5

Other Superficial Fungal Infections

Chapter 17: Candidiasis or Candidosis
Chapter 18: Pityriasis Versicolor
Chapter 19: Tinea Nigra Palmaris
Chapter 20: Piedra or Trichomycosis Nodularis

CHAPTER 17

Candidiasis or Candidosis

INTRODUCTION

Candidiasis refers to a range of superficial fungal infections of the skin, nail, and mucosae caused by yeasts belonging to the genus *Candida*. These infections can occur at any age, but certain age groups are more predisposed. These include extremes of age (neonates and elderly), childbearing age group, and with immunosuppression. There seems to be overall no sexual or racial predisposition.

The causative organisms belong to the genus *Candida* that includes approximately 200 species. The genus *Candida* is characterized by the formation of pseudohyphae with the exception of *Candida glabrata*. The most common species responsible for 70–80% of infection is *Candida albicans*. The species less frequently involved in mucocutaneous infection are *C. glabrata, Candida tropicalis, Candida krusei, Candida dubliniensis,* and *Candida parapsilosis.*

ETIOPATHOGENESIS

Candida albicans is often a normal inhabitant of the human gastrointestinal tract, vagina, and skin. The carriage rate for *C. albicans* in the gastrointestinal tract is almost 50–60%. In up to 20–25% of healthy asymptomatic women, *C. albicans* exists as a commensal in the vaginal mucosa. The yeast can also be occasionally isolated from the intertriginous areas. An increased skin pH, local occlusion and maceration, altered flora due to use of antibiotics, an impaired immune response in conditions like HIV, or presence of indwelling catheters favors candidal growth. The various predisposing factors are summarized in **Table 1**.

TABLE 1: Factors predisposing to the development of candidiasis.

Endocrine factors	Mechanical factors	Immunodeficiency	Iatrogenic factors
Diabetes	Local occlusion and high moisture levels causing maceration	Acquired immunodeficiency syndrome	Prolonged antibiotic use (disturbing the normal flora)
Cushing's syndrome	Obesity	DiGeorge's syndrome (defective T lymphocyte function)	Glucocorticoids
Pregnancy	Local tissue damage like burns, abrasions	Chronic granulomatous disease (defective macrophage function)	Oral contraceptives
Addison's disease		Myeloperoxidase deficiency (defective neutrophil function)	Immunosuppressives
Hypothyroidism		Severe combined immunodeficiency syndrome	
Hypoparathyroidism		Malignancy like leukemia and lymphomas	

CLINICAL FEATURES

Candidal infections produce very diverse cutaneous and mucosal manifestations depending on the area involved, the extent of disease, and host immunity. The clinical forms are summarized in **Box 1** and detailed below.

Oral Candidiasis

Oral cavity is one of the most common sites of *Candida* infection. The involvement of oral cavity can belong to any of the following clinical patterns.

Acute Pseudomembranous Candidiasis or Oral Thrush

Acute pseudomembranous candidiasis is the most common form of oral candidiasis. It is characterized by a grayish white semi-adherent membrane appearing in the buccal mucosa. It may present over the

BOX 1: Clinical manifestations of cutaneous candidal infections.

- *Oral candidiasis*:
  - Acute pseudomembranous candidiasis or oral thrush
  - Acute erythematous candidiasis (acute atrophic candidiasis)
  - Chronic pseudomembranous candidiasis
  - Chronic atrophic candidiasis (chronic erythematous candidiasis or denture stomatitis)
  - Angular cheilitis (Perlèche)
  - Chronic hyperplastic candidiasis
- Vaginal and vulvovaginal candidiasis (VVC)
- Candidal balanitis and balanoposthitis (CBP)
- Candidal intertrigo
- Perianal candidiasis
- Candidal paronychia
- Onychomycosis caused by *Candida*
- Diaper candidiasis or candidal diaper dermatitis
- Disseminated candidiasis
- Congenital candidiasis
- *Chronic mucocutaneous candidiasis (CMC)*:
  - Autosomal recessive CMC with endocrinopathy
  - Autosomal recessive CMC without endocrinopathy
  - Autosomal dominant CMC
  - Late-onset or thymoma-associated CMC
  - Idiopathic CMC

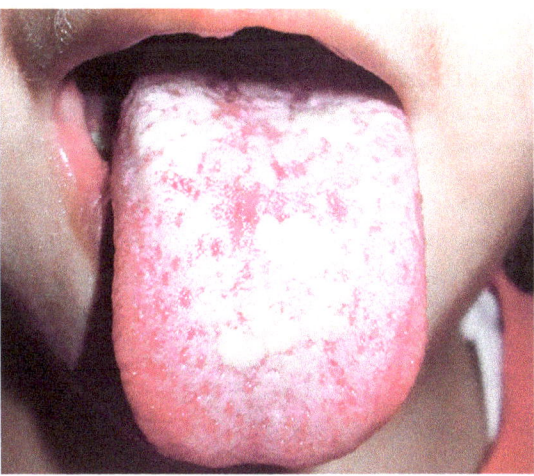

Fig. 1: Oral pseudomembranous candidiasis or thrush.

tongue, palate, or gingival area (**Fig. 1**). The base of these plaques is moist, red, and macerated. The grayish white membrane actually consists of desquamated epithelial cells, fungal elements, inflammatory cells, fibrin, and even food deposits. In immunosuppressed patients, the lesions may extend into the pharynx and esophagus causing odynophagia.

Differential Diagnosis

The differential diagnoses of oral thrush include common conditions like oral lichen planus, herpetic infection, erythema multiforme, or mucositis due to viral fever or chemotherapeutic agents.

Acute Erythematous Candidiasis (Acute Atrophic Candidiasis)

This condition is characterized by an atrophic, erythematous mucous membrane, especially involving the tongue. The clinical associations include the use of broad-spectrum antibiotic therapy, glucocorticoid usage, and HIV infection. The lesions are usually symptomatic, presenting with burning or pain.

Chronic Pseudomembranous Candidiasis

In this case, the lesions are morphologically similar to acute pseudomembranous candidiasis except that the lesions are more persistent.

Chronic Atrophic Candidiasis (Chronic Erythematous Candidiasis or Denture Stomatitis)

This condition is seen in 24–60% of denture wearers. It presents as chronic erythema and edema of the mucosa, especially the one coming in contact with dentures. Hence, it is commonly seen to involve the palate and gums. This pattern is often associated with angular cheilitis. Chronic mechanical irritation and occlusion are the two important factors in the *Candida* colonization.

Angular Cheilitis (Perlèche)

Perlèche presents as erythema, maceration, and fissuring at the oral commissures. The pattern of involvement is usually bilateral **(Fig. 2)**. This is a common presentation in habitual lip lickers. This condition can also be associated with the presence of coagulase-positive *Staphylococcus aureus* and gram-negative bacteria, apart from *Candida* infection.

Chronic Hyperplastic Candidiasis

This condition is more common in smokers characterized by thick, persistent, adherent white plaques on the tongue or cheek. This condition needs to be differentiated from the other causes of leukoplakia.

Vaginal and Vulvovaginal Candidiasis

Candidal vulvovaginitis is a common infection. Almost 75% of all women will experience at least one episode of VVC during their lifetime. The

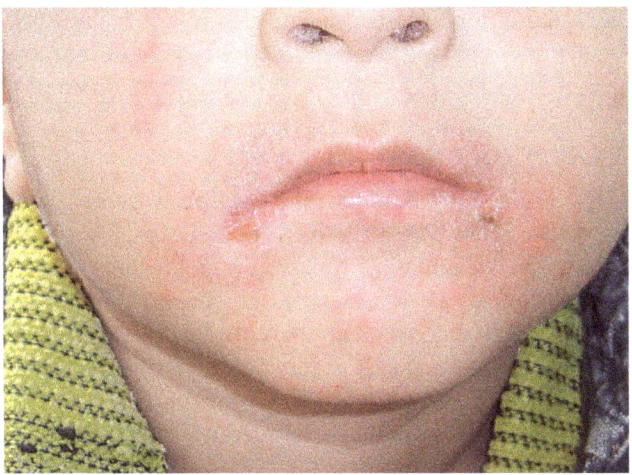

Fig. 2: Angular cheilitis in a young child.

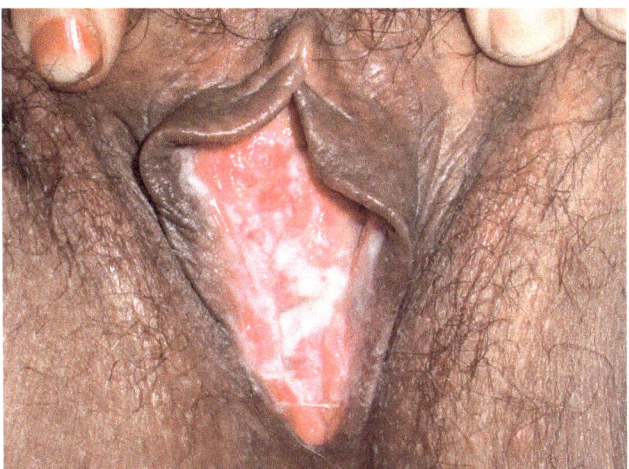

Fig. 3: Vulvovaginal candidiasis.

most common species involved is *C. albicans* accounting for 80-90% of cases followed by *C. glabrata*.

This condition presents as severe itching, burning, and thick white creamy discharge **(Fig. 3)**. Per speculum examination shows whitish plaques involving the vaginal walls. There is erythema and edema of the vaginal walls, and labia, extending even up to the perineum. In 5% of the cases, candidal vulvovaginitis may become recurrent (four or more symptomatic episodes per year).

Predisposing factors for vulvovaginal candidiasis include pregnancy, diabetes mellitus, broad-spectrum antibiotic usage, immunosuppression, obesity, steroid use, and tight-fitting synthetic undergarments.

Candidal Balanitis and Balanoposthitis

Candidal balanitis or balanoposthitis (CBP) is more common in uncircumcised sexually active males and in diabetics. It accounts for 30–35% cases of infective balanitis. This condition presents as tiny, fragile, papulopustules on the glans and prepuce. The lesions rupture to leave behind superficial erosions with a collarette of white scales **(Fig. 4)**. The presence of linear erosions is considered very characteristic of *Candida* etiology **(Fig. 5)**. In immunosuppressed patients, there may be severe inflammatory changes of the glans like edema and ulceration.

Candidal Intertrigo

Candidal intertrigo is the most common clinical presentation of candidiasis involving the glabrous skin. It can present as pruritic, pink to red, moist areas, associated with satellite vesicopustules. The sites commonly involved are the armpits, groins, intergluteal, interdigital, and submammary regions **(Figs. 6 and 7)**. The vesicopustules may rupture to leave behind collarette of white scales. In severe cases, there may be fissure formation.

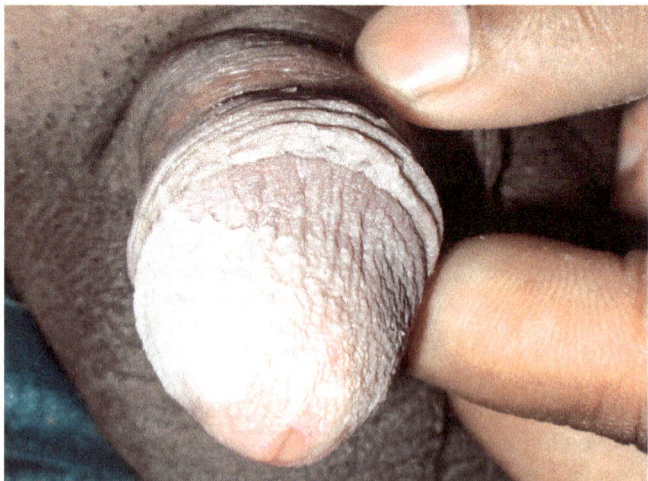

Fig. 4: Candidal balanoposthitis with characteristic white scale.

Differential Diagnosis

The differential diagnoses are summarized in **Box 2**. The important clinical differential diagnosis is tinea cruris, which is usually characterized by more scaliness and less maceration. The other close mimickers include erythrasma, bacterial intertrigo, flexural psoriasis, and seborrheic dermatitis.

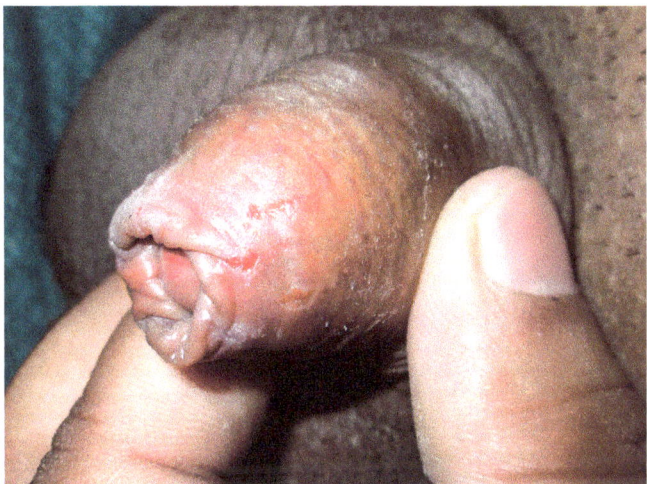

Fig. 5: Linear erosions over the glans are highly suggestive of candidal balanitis and balanoposthitis.

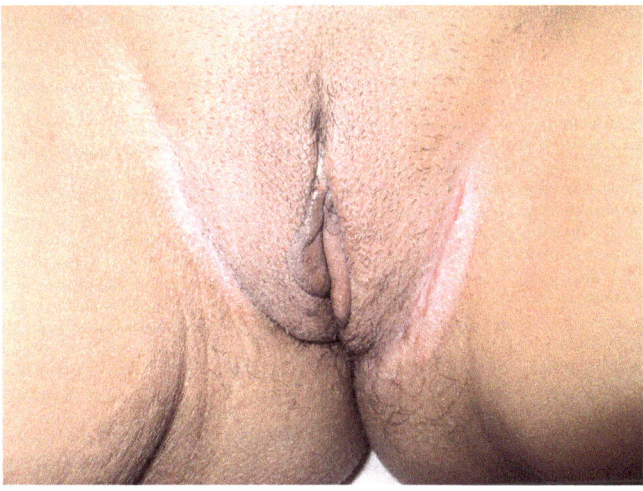

Fig. 6: Candidal intertrigo with erythema, scaling, and fissuring.

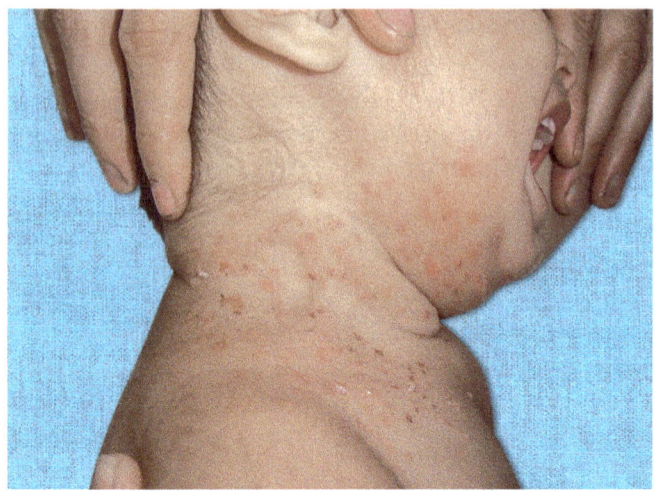

Fig. 7: Candidal intertrigo with characteristic satellite pustules.

BOX 2	Differential diagnosis of candidal intertrigo.
• Tinea cruris	• Flexural psoriasis
• Erythrasma	• Seborrheic dermatitis
• Bacterial intertrigo	

Perianal Candidiasis

Candidal infection in the intergluteal and perianal area may present as pruritis ani. It is characterized by redness, maceration, and oozing in the perianal region **(Fig. 8)**. Candidal superinfection may also be seen on pre-existing plaques of psoriasis or extramammary Paget's disease in this area.

Candidal Paronychia

Inflammation of the nail fold due to *Candida* is more common in housewives and food handlers who frequently immerse their hands in water. Apart from the yeast, bacterial coinfection and contact irritant dermatitis also play an important role. In early stages, there is redness, swelling, and tenderness of the proximal nail fold. Slowly, there is loss of cuticle and separation of proximal nail fold from nail

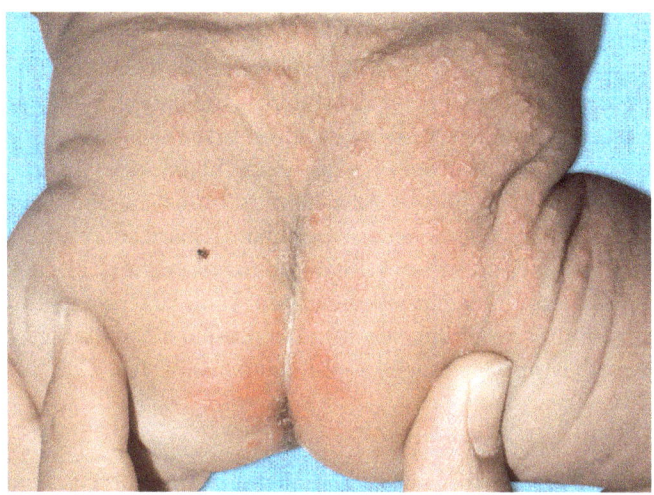

Fig. 8: Perianal candidiasis in a young child with characteristic satellite pustules.

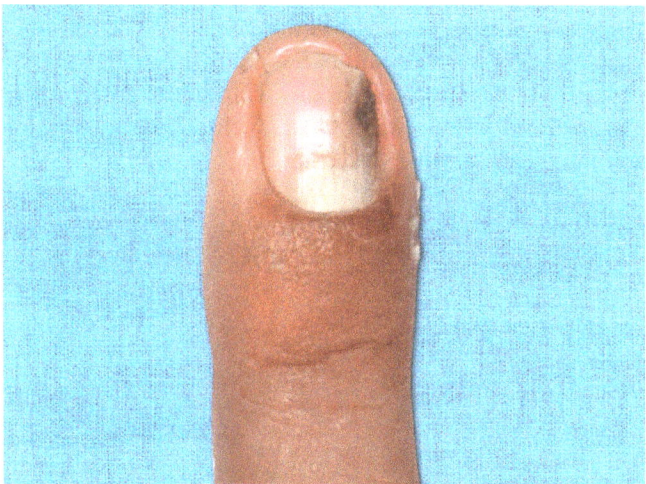

Fig. 9: Chronic paronychia with swelling and erythema of proximal and lateral nail fold. Note the absent to ragged cuticle and secondary nail dystrophy.

plate **(Fig. 9)**. In chronic cases, there is involvement of nail plate in the form of thickening and brownish discoloration, Beau's lines, distal onycholysis, and extensive nail damage in particularly long-standing cases. Avoidance of wet work is essential in the treatment.

Diaper Candidiasis or Candidal Diaper Dermatitis

Chronic occlusion caused by wet diapers creates ideal conditions for infection with *Candida* species derived from the patient's own gut flora. The condition is characterized by red, moist macules along with satellite pustules involving the borders in some cases. Rarely, after the resolution of diaper dermatitis, there is formation of brownish nodules on the buttocks, genitalia, upper thigh, and perineum. This occurs particularly in long-standing cases or in those with immunosuppression. This condition is known as "granuloma gluteale infantum" **(Fig. 10)**. Histopathology is diagnostic in this condition, showing the presence of a marked dermal infiltrate with lymphocytes, eosinophils, and histiocytes.

Disseminated Candidiasis

Candida can cause disseminated infection. The spread occurs via hematogenous route, especially in patients with compromised immunity. The predisposing factors include neutropenia, acquired immunodeficiency syndrome (AIDS), malnourished patients, transplant patients on immunosuppressive drugs, or a history of intravenous drug abuse. The infection involves multiple organs including skin. The skin lesions present as erythematous papules with central pustule distributed on the trunk and extremities. Patients also have fever and other constitutional symptoms like myalgias.

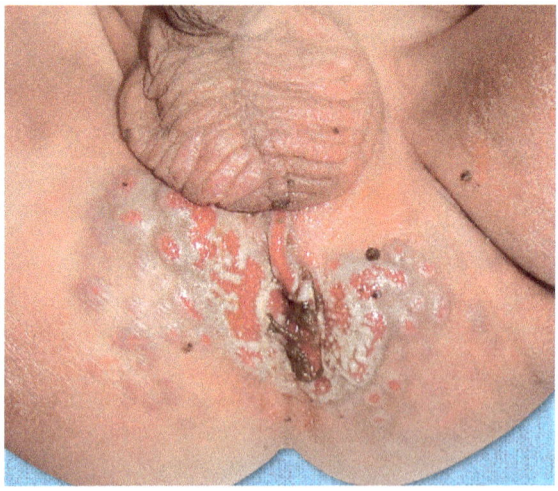

Fig. 10: Diaper involvement—granuloma gluteale infantum in a young child.

Congenital Candidiasis

Congenital candidiasis refers to a candidal infection of skin and mucous membranes presenting at the time of birth. This commonly occurs due to intrauterine transmission of the organism. The characteristic cutaneous lesions are discrete pustules on an erythematous base. In 10% cases, the infection may spread to the lungs or other organs. The condition needs to be differentiated from candidiasis of neonates occurring due to transmission of the organism from the birth canal during delivery.

Chronic Mucocutaneous Candidiasis

Chronic mucocutaneous candidiasis is a clinical syndrome characterized by persistent and recalcitrant candidal infection confined to the skin, nails, and mucous membrane. Although the clinical extent of involvement is generally massive, interestingly, invasive or disseminated candidiasis is not seen in this syndrome. The common feature is chronic noninvasive *Candida* infections of the skin, nails, and mucous membranes that are usually resistant to topical treatment, in the absence of invasive fungal infections.

Chronic mucocutaneous candidiasis can be either inherited or sporadic. The inherited variants may be associated with various polyendocrinopathies. Adult-onset cases are usually associated with a thymoma.

Etiopathogenesis

The patients with CMC generally have an underlying genetic or immune defect which makes them susceptible to acquiring *Candida* infection. CMC does not represent a specific disease but rather a phenotypic presentation of a spectrum of immunologic, endocrinologic, and autoimmune disorders. The unifying feature of these heterogeneous disorders is an impaired cell-mediated immunity against *Candida* species. Various mechanisms have been postulated including an impaired production of IL-12, IL-17 receptor mutation, decreased number of natural killer (NK) cells, decreased serum intracellular adhesion molecules (ICAM1), or increased levels of IL-6 and IL-10.

Epidemiology

The onset of disease is usually before the age of 6 years. The male-to-female ratio is equal. There is no sex predilection. CMC is not associated with high-degree mortality.

Clinical Features

The main clinical manifestations are persistent oral thrush, angular cheilitis or perlèche, esophageal or genital candidiasis, chronic paronychia, and total dystrophic onychomycosis (TDO). Skin involvement can occur most often in the form of candidal intertrigo, though sometimes lesions may spread to involve the trunk and limbs. Apart from increased susceptibility to *Candida*, the patients may also develop other skin infections like dermatophytosis and warts. CMC may include several clinical syndromes described as follows:

- *Autosomal recessive CMC with endocrinopathy*, also known as autoimmune polyendocrinopathy candidiasis ectodermal dystrophy (APECED). Its onset is usually in childhood and it is associated with other features like hypoparathyroidism, hypoadrenalism, hypothyroidism, or polyendocrinopathy. Recently, this syndrome has been linked to mutation in chromosome 2p. The patient may also manifest other associated autoimmune disorders like alopecia areata, vitiligo, pernicious anemia, and type 1 diabetes mellitus.
- *Autosomal recessive CMC without endocrinopathy* manifests usually in the first decade with persistent oral and nail involvement. The skin involvement is less common. These patients may improve with advancing age.
- *Autosomal dominant CMC* also manifests in childhood like autosomal recessive variant, though involvement can be more severe.
- *Late-onset or thymoma-associated CMC* is sporadic and has onset in adulthood (after the third decade). The CMC manifests often before the onset of thymoma. The patient may also have features of myasthenia gravis.
- *Idiopathic CMC* is a subgroup of severely affected patients with candidal granuloma formation and associated bronchiectasis and pulmonary bullae. The candidal granuloma formation is due to inability of neutrophils and macrophages to ingest the yeast cells. On histopathological examination, there is hyperkeratosis, papillomatosis along with dermal infiltration by lymphocytes and multinucleate giant cells.

DIAGNOSIS

The confirmation of diagnosis of candidiasis is simply by demonstration of typical budding yeast cells (2–6 µm × 3–9 µm) **(Fig. 11)** with narrow base accompanied by hyphae or pseudohyphae (except for *C. glabrata*)

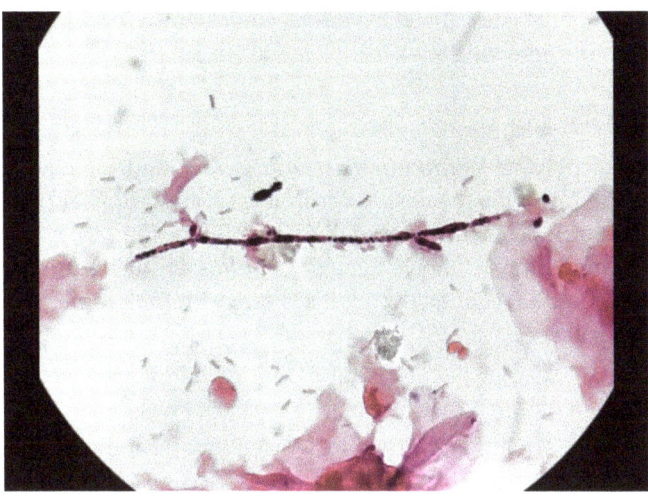

Fig. 11: *Candida* pseudohyphae and budding yeasts (KOH mount 400×).

by light microscopy. *C. albicans* grows easily on cycloheximide-free culture media [Sabouraud's dextrose agar (SDA)] at 37°C; whitish mucoid colonies appear in 2–5 days. However, the plate should be incubated for 1 week before reporting it as negative. CHROMagar *Candida* is a new medium that is used for isolation and identification of some clinically important species and can differentiate between different species on the basis of color produced by the fungal colonies. It is important to identify the species implicated, as some nonalbicans species like *C. glabrata* and *C. krusei* show primary fluconazole resistance. The characteristic feature of *C. albicans* is the ability to produce germ tubes when incubated in serum at 37°C for 2–4 hours. The only other species that can produce germ tube is *C. dubliniensis*, known to cause oral thrush in HIV-positive patients. Histopathology from the satellite pustule shows subcorneal neutrophil accumulation. The yeast cells can be demonstrated in stratum corneum with periodic acid–Schiff (PAS) stain or methenamine silver stain. In disseminated candidiasis, the organism is seen inside the blood vessels by special stains.

TREATMENT

Apart from specific therapy for candidiasis, it is important to treat or alter the underlying predisposing factors like diabetes mellitus, Addison's disease, Cushing's syndrome, or other causes of immunosuppression.

The treatment measures used in various clinical forms of candidiasis are detailed in the following text:

Topical Therapy

The topical polyene compound *nystatin* is safe and effective against most of the *Candida* species. Apart from polyenes, topical imidazoles like miconazole, clotrimazole, and econazole are the other important group of antifungals effective against *Candida* and without significant resistance. Contact allergic dermatitis is rare with both topical polyenes and imidazoles.

Systemic Therapy

The systemic treatment measures used for Candidal infections are summarized in **Table 2**. This includes drugs like ketoconazole, fluconazole, and itraconazole, which have significant anticandidal action. The major adverse effect of ketoconazole is hepatotoxicity, which is uncommon with fluconazole and itraconazole. The usual doses of ketoconazole, fluconazole, and itraconazole are 200, 100–400, and 200–400 mg, respectively. Intravenous liposomal amphotericin B and fluconazole can be used for disseminated candidiasis.

TABLE 2: Oral treatment options for various clinical types of cutaneous candidiasis.

Indication	Drug	Dosage	Duration of therapy
Oropharyngeal candidiasis	Itraconazole	100 mg OD	7 days
	Fluconazole	100–200 mg OD	7 days
Vulvovaginal candidiasis	Itraconazole	600 mg stat	Single dose
	Fluconazole	150 mg stat	Single dose
Recurrent vulvovaginal candidiasis	Fluconazole	150 mg on 0, 3, 7 days; then 150 mg/wk for 6 months	
Candidal onychomycosis	Itraconazole	200 mg BD for 7 days in a month (one cycle)	2–3 cycles
	Fluconazole	300 mg/week	4 weeks for finger nails and 12 weeks for toenails

(OD: once a day; BD: twice daily)

Oral Candidiasis

General measures like maintenance of good oral hygiene and removal of dentures at night are important. Therapy could include topical nystatin suspension (4,00,000-6,00,000 units) applied four times a day or clotrimazole mouth paint applied five times a day. These are reported to be effective in cases with acute pseudomembranous candidiasis. This condition usually responds to treatment in 10-14 days. For chronic and severe cases like hyperplastic or atrophic candidiasis, oral antifungals are warranted. These could be either fluconazole (100-200 mg/day) or itraconazole (100-200 mg/day). If the lesions do not respond to a fair trial of oral antifungals, it is necessary to consider histopathology to differentiate from other causes of leukoplakia.

Genital Candidiasis

The recommended treatment for genital candidiasis is a single 150 mg dose of fluconazole along with topical imidazoles in the form of intravaginal pessaries or creams. In case of recurrent VVC, a weekly fluconazole 150 mg tablet orally or clotrimazole 500 mg tablet intravaginally can be used effectively.

Candidal Intertrigo

Intertriginous *Candida* responds to topical azoles or polyenes in approximately 2 weeks. The powder formulations can be used to keep the affected region dry. In case of no response, it is important to rule out bacterial intertrigo, flexural psoriasis, or seborrheic dermatitis.

Candidal Paronychia and Onychomycosis

Prolonged topical antifungal treatment is required in cases of chronic paronychia, in addition to minimizing the wet work. Sometimes, topical corticosteroid can be added to topical antifungals in cases of suspected contact allergic or irritant dermatitis. In proven cases of candidal onychomycosis, oral fluconazole and itraconazole can be used successfully. Itraconazole can be used as continuous or pulse regimen. Fluconazole is given as 50 mg/day or 300 mg/wk to be continued for minimum 4 weeks for fingernail and 12 weeks for toenail onychomycosis.

Chronic Mucocutaneous Candidiasis

Prolonged and repeated courses of oral antifungals like fluconazole and itraconazole, given at doses higher than usual, are generally needed for these cases. Maintenance therapy needs to be avoided to prevent the development of resistance. Endocrine screening test and serum iron levels should also be done repeatedly, as endocrine dysfunction may manifest years after the first occurrence of candidiasis.

CHAPTER 18

Pityriasis Versicolor

INTRODUCTION

It is a chronic infection of the stratum corneum caused by *Malassezia* species. It is characterized by hypopigmented or hyperpigmented coalescing scaly macules over the trunk. The condition is also known as *tinea versicolor*. The disease is more common in teenagers and young adults with no sexual predilection. Infants can also develop skin lesions that occur more commonly on the face. The disease is more commonly seen in hot and humid climate.

ETIOPATHOGENESIS

The genus *Malassezia* includes at least 12 species of lipophilic yeast: *M. furfur*, *M. pachydermatis* (does not require exogenous lipids), *M. sympodialis* (part of normal flora of human skin), *M. globosa* (most frequently associated with clinical disease), *M. restricta*, *M. obtusa*, *M. dermatis*, *M. equi*, *M. slooffi*, *M. japonica*, *M. yamotoensis*, and *M. nana* are the isolated species. The yeast form of the organism is a part of the resident flora, whereas the hyphal phase is implicated in producing the skin lesions. The predisposing factors for the infection are multiple and include genetic susceptibility, tropical climate, Cushing's syndrome, malnutrition, and excessive sebum production.

CLINICAL FEATURES

The most common presentation is in the form of hypopigmented or hyperpigmented coalescing macules. These have a characteristic furfuraceous or fine branny scale **(Figs. 1 and 2)**. The scale can be demonstrated better on lightly scratching the skin (scratch sign). The sites of predilection are the sternal region, sides of the chest, upper arms, abdomen, back and neck, and intertriginous areas. The patients are usually asymptomatic.

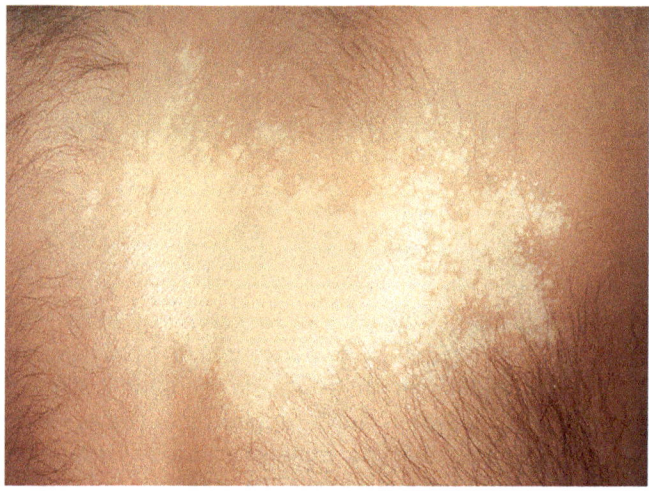

Fig. 1: Pityriasis versicolor (hypopigmented variant). The lesions can be isolated or confluent. Mild scaling can be appreciated.

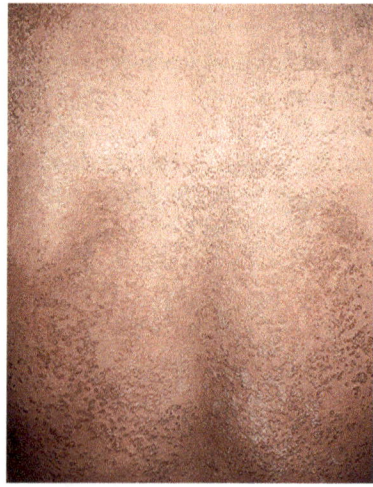

Fig. 2: Pityriasis versicolor (hyperpigmented variant). The lesions can be isolated or confluent. Mild scaling can be appreciated.

The characteristic hypopigmentation seen in the disease is due to abnormally small and poorly melanized melanosomes; production of dicarboxylic acids such as azelaic acid by the fungus, which cause competitive inhibition of tyrosinase enzyme; and the presence of pityriacitrin compound that absorbs ultraviolet (UV) light. The hyperpigmented skin lesions are postulated to be due to abnormally large melanosomes.

DIAGNOSIS

Direct microscopic examination of the lesional scrapings is generally sufficient to establish the diagnosis. The fungus can be easily demonstrated in KOH mount of scale scraped from the lesions. A combination of mycelium (2–5 µm wide and 25 µm long) with spherical thick-walled yeasts (2–8 µm wide) commonly referred to as "spaghetti and meatballs" or "banana and grapes" appearance confirms the diagnosis **(Fig. 3)**. The organism can also be cultured in lipid-enriched media but this is rarely resorted to in clinical practice. Wood's lamp examination may show yellow fluorescence of involved skin.

DIFFERENTIAL DIAGNOSIS

The differential diagnoses are summarized in **Box 1**.

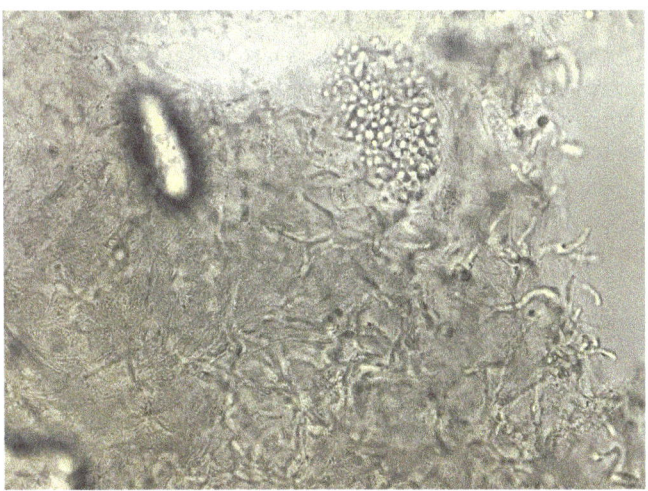

Fig. 3: Spaghetti and meatballs appearance (KOH mount 400×).
(KOH: potassium hydroxide)

BOX 1	Differential diagnosis of pityriasis versicolor.
• Pityriasis alba • Pityriasis rosea • Seborrheic dermatitis	• Tinea infection • Secondary syphilis (always rule out) • Vitiligo • Erythrasma • Psoriasis • Pityriasis rubra pilaris

TABLE 1: Treatment options for pityriasis versicolor.

Topical	Systemic
Selenium sulfide 2.5% shampoo (left on for at least 10 minutes) for 14 days	Ketoconazole 400 mg stat or 200 mg daily for 7 days
Ketoconazole 2% shampoo (left for 5 minutes) for 3 days	Itraconazole 200 mg daily for 7 days or 400 mg stat
Terbinafine 1% cream BD for 14 days	Fluconazole 400 mg stat

(BD: twice daily)

TREATMENT

Various topical and systemic antifungal agents can be used for the treatment of tinea versicolor. These are summarized in **Table 1**. The most commonly used drugs are azole antifungals and the usual time to recovery is 2-3 weeks. The patients must be counseled that hypopigmentation may take further 2-3 months to resolve. Relapses are, however, very common. A comparative trial concluded that a single dose of fluconazole 400 mg is associated with the lowest risk of relapse at 12 months. General measures such as wearing nonocclusive clothing and avoiding excessive sweating, help in reducing the risk of further relapse.

PREVENTION

Oral antifungals used in prophylactic doses can be effective in decreasing the chances of a relapse. Oral ketoconazole 400 mg or fluconazole 400 mg can be repeated at monthly intervals for the same. Similarly, topical antifungal shampoos or zinc pyrithione bar have also been used to avoid relapse.

OTHER CUTANEOUS DISORDERS ASSOCIATED WITH *MALASSEZIA*

The *Malassezia* yeasts have also been associated with other skin conditions such as confluent and reticulate papillomatosis, acne vulgaris, seborrheic dermatitis, sebopsoriasis and pulmonary and systemic infections in infants on long-term intravenous lipid therapy. Among these, the commonly seen manifestation is Pityrosporum (*Malassezia*) folliculitis. The typical lesions of Pityrosporum folliculitis are moderately itchy dome-shaped follicular papules involving upper back and adjacent areas **(Fig. 4)**. It is most often seen in adolescent males. The condition usually responds to topical and systemic antifungals as mentioned above. Relapses are common and can be prevented by monthly application of selenium sulfide or maintenance doses of oral azole antifungals.

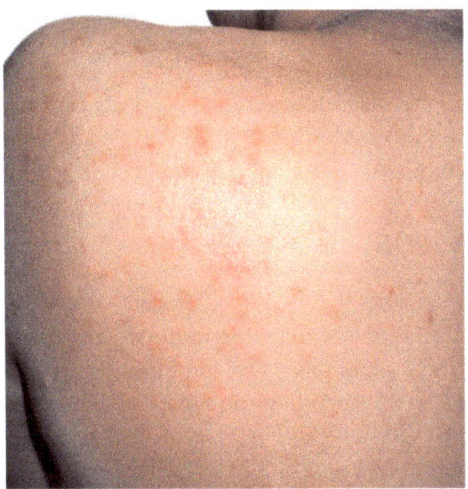

Fig. 4: Pityrosporum folliculitis in a young male.

CHAPTER 19

Tinea Nigra Palmaris

INTRODUCTION

Tinea nigra is the superficial infection of the stratum corneum caused by *Exophiala werneckii* or *Hortaea werneckii*. The condition predominantly affects the palms. Hence, it is also known as pityriasis nigra and keratomycosis nigricans palmaris. Tinea nigra is reported from tropical and subtropical areas including central and South America, Asia, and Australia. It has a distinct female predilection (F:M = 3:1).

ETIOPATHOGENESIS

The causative organism *Exophiala werneckii* or *Hortaea werneckii* is black-colored yeast that is widely distributed in hot and humid climates. The fungus is directly inoculated by trauma into the stratum corneum. The infection has an incubation period of 2–7 weeks.

CLINICAL FEATURES

It presents as one or several asymptomatic brown or black macules predominantly on the palms with minimal or no scaling. Other less commonly involved sites are soles, neck, and rarely trunk. Spontaneous resolution is generally not seen.

DIAGNOSIS

Potassium hydroxide (KOH) mount reveals abundant brown-colored, thick, branching, closely septate hyphae (up to 5 μm in diameter) along with oval-to-spindle-shaped yeast cells. Culture can be done on Sabouraud dextrose agar which reveals the presence of glossy black colonies within 1 week. Dermatoscopy has also been reported to be useful in differentiating this infection from a melanocytic lesion.

DIFFERENTIAL DIAGNOSIS

The differential diagnoses are summarized in **Box 1**.

> **BOX 1**   **Differential diagnosis of tinea nigra palmaris.**
> - Junctional nevus
> - Syphilis
> - Pinta
> - Addison's disease
> - Chemical exposure

TREATMENT

Tinea nigra responds to topical antifungals such as clotrimazole, miconazole, ketoconazole, econazole, and terbinafine. Topical keratolytic agents such as salicylic acid ointment have also been used effectively. Treatment should be continued for 2–4 weeks after the clinical resolution to prevent relapse. Systemic therapies are not usually indicated.

CHAPTER 20

Piedra or Trichomycosis Nodularis

INTRODUCTION

It is a superficial fungal infection of the hair shaft, also known as trichomycosis nodularis. Black piedra is more commonly seen in tropical countries with hot humid climate. It can affect both human as well as primate's hair shaft. White piedra is more common in temperate climate.

ETIOPATHOGENESIS

Black piedra is caused by *Piedraia hortae* while white piedra is caused by pathogenic species of *Trichosporon beigelii*.

CLINICAL FEATURES

Black piedra is characterized by the presence of multiple, firmly adherent, dark, pinhead sized, hard nodules on the hair of scalp or less frequently brows, lashes, beard, or pubic hair **(Fig. 1)**. The fungus may enter into the hair shaft causing its fracture.

White piedra presents with multiple, white- or beige-colored soft, less adherent nodules. It is more common in beard, moustache, and pubic hair. The broken stump of hair can be seen but less common than in black piedra.

DIAGNOSIS

The nodules can be seen adhering to the hair shaft on trichoscopy **(Fig. 2)**. After removal and dissolution in KOH, the nodules of black piedra show brown septate hyphae along with chlamydoconidia.

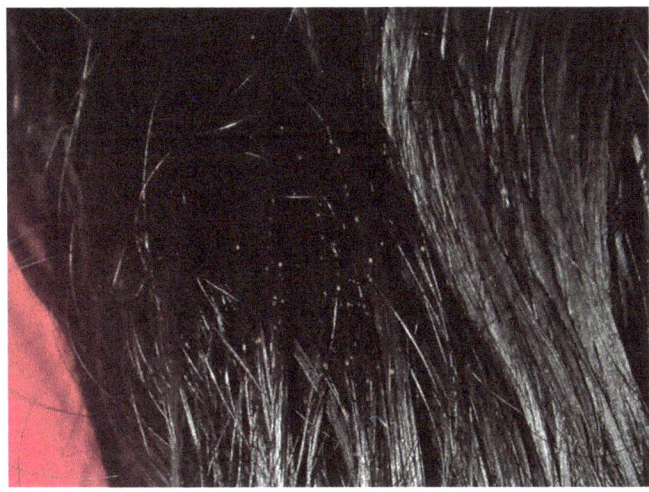

Fig. 1: Piedra in long hair. Note the barely visible dark brown concretions attached to the hair shaft along its length. The concretions can be made more visible by wetting the hair.

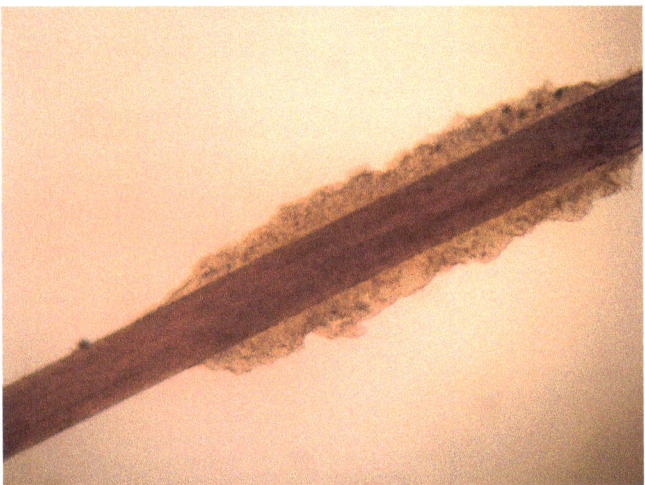

Fig. 2: Dermascopic image showing piedra nodules adherent to the hair shaft (100×).

The fungus can be grown in Sabouraud dextrose agar (SDA) with cycloheximide to form black colonies. While the white piedra nodules demonstrate hyphae, arthroconidia, and budding cells under KOH examination. *Trichosporon* can be grown in SDA and is inhibited by cycloheximide.

DIFFERENTIAL DIAGNOSIS

The differential diagnoses are summarized in **Box 1**.

BOX 1	Differential diagnosis of piedra or trichomycosis nodularis.

- Nits
- Hair casts or pilar casts

TREATMENT

Cutting or shaving the infected hair shaft is the simple and curative treatment modality for both black and white piedra. Various topical as well as systemic antifungals have been reported to have low efficacy such as topical imidazoles, ciclopirox, selenium sulfide 2%, oral antifungals such as itraconazole and terbinafine at least for 6–8 weeks.

Bibliography

1. Akilov OE, Mumcuoglu KY. Immune response in demodicosis. J Eur Acad Dermatol Venereol. 2004;18(4):440-4.
2. Antonsson A, Forslund O, Ekberg H, Sterner G, Hansson BG. The ubiquity and impressive genomic diversity of human skin papillomaviruses suggest a commensalic nature of these viruses. J Virol. 2000;74:11636-41.
3. Armstrong-Esther CA, Smith JE. Carriage patterns of Staphylococcus aureus in a healthy non-hospital population of adults and children. Ann Hum Biol. 1976;3:221-7.
4. Astori G, Lavergne D, Benton C, Höckmayr B, Egawa K, Garbe C, et al. Human papillomaviruses are commonly found in normal skin of immunocompetent hosts. J Invest Dermatol. 1998;110:752-5.
5. Aylesworth R, Vance JC. Demodex folliculorum and Demodex brevis in cutaneous biopsies. J Am Acad Dermatol. 1982;7(5):583-9.
6. Balakumar S, Rajan S. Epidemiology of dermatophytosis in and around Tiruchirapalli, Tamilnadu, India. Asian Pac J Trop Dis. 2012;2(4):286-8.
7. Barth JH. Nasal carriage of staphylococci and streptococci. Int J Dermatol. 1987;26:24-6.
8. Basta-Juzbasic´ A, Subic´ JS, Ljubojevic´ S. Demodex folliculorum in development of dermatitis rosaceiformis steroidica and rosacea-related diseases. Clin Dermatol. 2002;20(2):135-40.
9. Batta K, Ramlogan D, Smith AG, Garrido MC, Moss C. 'Tinea indecisiva' may mimic the concentric rings of tinea imbricata. Br J Dermatol. 2002;147(2):384.
10. Bhat YJ, Keen A, Hassan I, Latif I, Bashir S. Can dermoscopy serve as a diagnostic tool in dermatophytosis? A pilot study. Indian Dermatol Online J. 2019;10(5):530-5.
11. Bishnoi A, Vinay K, Dogra S. Emergence of recalcitrant dermatophytosis in India. Lancet Infect Dis. 2018;18(3):250-1.
12. Capone KA, Dowd SE, Stamatas GN, Nikolovski J. Diversity of the human skin microbiome early in life. J Invest Dermatol. 2011;131:2026-32.
13. Castriota M, Ricci F, Paradisi A, Simone CD, Capizzi R, Guerriero C. Erythema nodosum induced by kerion celsi of the scalp in a child: a case report and mini-review of literature. Mycoses. 2013;56(3):200-3.
14. Chander J. Dermatophytoses. Textbook of Medical Mycology. New Delhi: Jaypee Brothers Medical Publishers (P) Ltd.; 1995. pp. 91-112.
15. Chen YE, Tsao H. The skin microbiome: current perspectives and future challenges. J Am Acad Dermatol. 2013;69(1):143-55.
16. Cogen AL, Yamasaki K, Muto J, Sanchez KM, Alexander LC, Tanios J, et al. *Staphylococcus epidermidis* antimicrobial delta-toxin (phenol-soluble modulin-gamma) cooperates with host antimicrobial peptides to kill group A *Streptococcus*. PLoS One. 2010;5:e8557.
17. Costello EK, Lauber CL, Hamady M, Fierer N, Gordon JI, Knight R. Bacterial community variation in human body habitats across space and time. Science. 2009;326:1694-7.
18. Debh V. Studies in medical mycology: Part one. Incidence of dermatomycosis in Warangal, AP (India). Indian J Med Res. 1965;54:468.
19. Dominguez-Bello MG, Costello EK, Contreras M, Magris M, Hidalgo G, Fie*rer* N, et al. *Delivery* mode shapes the acquisition and structure of the initial microbiota across multiple body habitats in newborns. Proc Natl Acad Sci USA. 2010;107:11971-5.

20. Drake TE, Maibach HI. Candida and candidiasis. Cultural conditions, epidemiology and pathogenesis. Postgrad Med. 1973;53(2):83-7.
21. Dréno B, Pécastaings S, Corvec S, Veraldi S, Khammari A, Roques C. Cutibacterium acnes (Propionibacterium acnes) and acne vulgaris: a brief look at the latest updates. J Eur Acad Dermatol Venereol. 2018;32(Suppl 2):5-14.
22. Elewski BE. Treatment of tinea capitis: beyond griseofulvin. J Am Acad Dermatol. 1999;40(6 Pt 2): S27-30.
23. Emmons CW. Dermatophytes: natural groupings based on the form of the spores and accessory organs. Arch Dermatol Syphilol. 1934;30:337-62.
24. Forton F, Seys B. Density of Demodex folliculorum in rosacea: a case-control study using standardized skin-surface biopsy. Br J Dermatol. 1993;128(6):650-9.
25. Forton F, Song M. Limitations of standardized skin surface biopsy in measurement of the density of Demodex folliculorum. A case report. Br J Dermatol. 1998;139(4):697-700.
26. Foulongne V, Sauvage V, Hebert C, Dereure O, Cheval J, Gouilh MA, et al. Human skin microbiota: high diversity of DNA viruses identified on the human skin by high throughput sequencing. PLoS ONE. 2012;7:e38499.
27. Gallo RL, Nakatsuji T. Microbial symbiosis with the innate immune defense system of the skin. J Invest Dermatol. 2011;131:1974-80.
28. Ghannoum M, Isham N, Hajjeh R, Cano M, Al-Hasawi F, Yearick D, et al. Tinea capitis in Cleveland: Survey of elementary school students. J Am Acad Dermatol. 2003;48(2):189-93.
29. Grice EA, Kong HH, Renaud G, Young AC; NISC Comparative Sequencing Program; Bouffard GG, Blakesley RW, et al. A diversity profile of the human skin microbiota. Genome Res. 2008;18:1043-50.
30. Grover C, Arora P, Manchanda V. Comparative evaluation of griseofulvin, terbinafine and fluconazole in the treatment of tinea capitis. Int J Dermatol. 2012;51(4):455-8.
31. Grover C, Arora P, Manchanda V. Tinea capitis in the pediatric population: a study from North India. Indian J Dermatol Venereol Leprol. 2010;76(5):527-32.
32. Grover C, Khurana A. Onychomycosis: newer insights in pathogenesis and diagnosis. Indian J Dermatol Venereol Leprol. 2012;78(3):263-70.
33. Grover C, Reddy BS, Chaturvedi KU. Onychomycosis and the diagnostic significance of nail biopsy. J Dermatol. 2003;30(2):116-22.
34. Hamory BH, Parisi JT. *Staphylococcus epidermidis*: a significant nosocomial pathogen. Am J Infect Control. 1987;15:59-74.
35. Haneke E, Roseeuw D. The scope of onychomycosis: epidemiology and clinical features. Int J Dermatol. 1999;38:7-12.
36. Hay RJ, Baran R. Onychomycosis: a proposed revision of the clinical classification. J Am Acad Dermatol. 2011;65(6):1219-27.
37. Hay RJ, Shennan G. Chronic dermatophyte infections II. Antibody and cell mediated immune responses. Br J Dermatol. 1982;106:191-5.
38. Kalla G, Begra B, Solanki A, Goyal A, Batra A. Clinicomycological study of tinea capitis in desert district of Rajasthan. Indian J Dermatol Venereol Leprol. 1995;61:342-5.
39. Karincaoglu Y, Bayram N, Aycan O, Esrefoglu M. The clinical importance of demodex folliculorum presenting with nonspecific facial signs and symptoms. J Dermatol. 2004;31(8):618-26.
40. Kligman AM, Leyden JJ, McGinley KJ. Bacteriology. J Invest Dermatol. 1976;67:160-8.
41. Kloos WE. The identification of *Staphylococcus* and *Micrococcus* species isolated from human skin. In: Maibach H, Aly R (Eds). Skin Microbiology: Relevance to Clinical Infection. New York: Springer-Verlag; 1981. pp. 3-12.
42. Lambkin E, Hamilton A, Hay RJ. Partial purification and characterization of a 235,000 Mr extracellular proteinase from Trichophyton rubrum. Mycoses. 1994;37:85-92.

43. Looming JP, Holland KT, Cunliffe WJ. The microbial ecology of pilosebaeous units isolated from human skin. J Gen Microbiol. 1984;130:803-7.
44. Michaels BD, Del Rosso JQ. Tinea capitis in infants: recognition, evaluation, and management suggestions. J Clin Aesthet Dermatol. 2012;5(2):49-59.
45. Moens U, Ludvigsen M, Van Ghelue M. Human polyomaviruses in skin diseases. Patholog Res Int. 2011;2011:123491.
46. Nagabhushanum P, Singh N, Patniak R. Tinea capitis in Hyderabad. Indian J Dermatol Venereol Leprosy. 1972;30:26-9.
47. Nakaminami H, Noguchi N, Nishijima S, Kurokawa I, So H, Sasatsu M. Transduction of the plasmid encoding antiseptic resistance gene qacB in *Staphylococcus aureus*. Biol Pharm Bull. 2007;30:1412-5.
48. Nenoff P, Verma SB, Uhrlaß S, Burmester A, Gräser Y. A clarion call for preventing taxonomical errors of dermatophytes using the example of the novel Trichophyton mentagrophytes genotype VIII uniformly isolated in the Indian epidemic of superficial dermatophytosis. Mycoses. 2019;62:6-10.
49. Noble WC. Microbiology of Human Skin. London: Lloyd-Luke; 1981.
50. Noble WC. Skin microbiology: coming of age. J Med Microbiol. 1984;17:1-12.
51. Okyay P, Ertabaklar H, Savk E, Erfug S. Prevalence of Demodex folliculorum in young adults: relation with sociodemographic/hygienic factors and acne vulgaris. J Eur Acad Dermatol Venereol. 2006;20(4):474-6.
52. Pallotta S, Cianchini G, Martelloni E, Ferranti G, Girardelli CR, Di Lella G, et al. Unilateral demodicidosis. Eur J Dermatol. 1998;8(3):191-2.
53. Panda S, Verma S. The menace of dermatophytosis in India: The evidence that we need. Indian J Dermatol Venereol Leprol. 2017;83:281-284.
54. Peck SM. Fungus antigens and their importance as sensitizers in the general population. Ann NY Acad Sci. 1950;50:1362-5.
55. Price PB. The bacteriology of normal skin: a new quantitative test applied to a study of the bacterial flora and the disinfectant action of mechanical cleansing. J Infect Dis. 1938;63:301-18.
56. Rajagopalan M, Inamadar A, Mittal A, Miskeen AK, Srinivas CR, Sardana K, et al. Expert Consensus on The Management of Dermatophytosis in India (ECTODERM India). BMC Dermatol. 2018;18(1):6.
57. Rao AG, Datta N. Tinea corporis due to Trichophyton mentagrophytes and Trichophyton tonsurans mimicking tinea imbricata. Indian J Dermatol Venereol Leprol. 2013;79(4):554.
58. Ray A, Singh BS, Kar BR. Clinicomycological Profile of Pediatric Dermatophytoses: An Observational Study. Indian Dermatol Online J. 2022 May 5;13(3):361-5.
59. Retailliau HF, Hightower AW, Dixon RE, Allen JR. Acinetobacter calcoaceticus: a nosocomial pathogen with an unusual seasonal pattern. J Infect Dis. 1979;139:371-5.
60. Rubenstein RM, Malerich SA. Malassezia (pityrosporum) folliculitis. J Clin Aesthet Dermatol. 2014;7(3):37-41.
61. Saraswat A, Lahiri K, Chatterjee M, Barua S, Coondoo A, Mittal A, et al. Topical corticosteroid abuse on the face: a prospective, multicenter study of dermatology outpatients. Indian J Dermatol Venereol Leprol. 2011;77:160-6.
62. Sarkany I, Gaylarde CC. Bacterial colonization of the skin of the newborn. J Pathol Bacteriol. 1968;95:115-22.
63. Schowalter RM, Pastrana DV, Pumphrey KA, Moyer AL, Buck CB. Merkel cell polyomavirus and two previously unknown polyomaviruses are chronically shed from human skin. Cell Host Microbe. 2010;7:509-15.
64. Singal A, Rawat S, Bhattacharya SN, Mohanty S, Baruah MC. Clinico-mycological profile of tinea capitis in North India and response to griseofulvin. J Dermatol. 2001;28(1):22-6.

65. Singh S, Beena PM. Profile of dermatophyte infections in Baroda. Indian J Dermatol Venereol Leprol. 2003;69(4):281-3.
66. Somerville-Millar DA, Noble WC. Resident and transient bacteria of the skin. J Cutan Pathol. 1974;1:260-4.
67. Somerville DA. Erythrasma in normal young adults. J Med Microbiol. 1970;3:352-6.
68. Tainwala R, Sharma Y. Pathogenesis of dermatophytoses. Indian J Dermatol. 2011;56(3): 259-61.
69. Uehara Y, Kikuchi K, Nakamura T, Nakama H, Agematsu K, Kawakami Y, et al. Inhibition of methicillin-resistant *Staphylococcus aureus* colonization of oral cavities in newborns by viridans group streptococci. Clin Infect Dis. 2001;32:1399-407.
70. Uehara Y, Nakama H, Agematsu K, Uchida M, Kawakami Y, Abdul Fattah AS, et al. Bacterial interference among nasal inhabitants: eradication of *Staphylococcus aureus* from nasal cavities by artificial implantation of Corynebacterium sp. J Hosp Infect. 2000;44:127-33.
71. Uhrlaß S, Verma SB, Gräser Y, Rezaei-Matehkolaei A, Hatami M, Schaller M, et al. *Trichophyton indotineae*—An emerging pathogen causing recalcitrant dermatophytoses in india and worldwide—A multidimensional perspective. J Fungi (Basel). 2022;8(7):757.
72. Umborowati MA, Damayanti D, Anggraeni S, Endaryanto A, Surono IS, Effendy I, et al. The role of probiotics in the treatment of adult atopic dermatitis: a meta-analysis of randomized controlled trials. J Health Popul Nutr. 2022;41(1):37.
73. Varga M, Kuntova L, Pantucek R, Mašlaňová I, Růžičková V, Doškař J. Efficient transfer of antibiotic resistance plasmids by transduction within methicillin-resistant *Staphylococcus aureus USA300 clone*. FEMS Microbiol Lett. 2012;332:146-52.
74. Verma S, Vasani R, Reszke R, Matusiak L, Szepietowski JC. The influence of superficial dermatophytoses epidemic in India on patients' quality of life. Postepy Dermatol Alergol. 2021;38(2):102-105.
75. Verma SB, Panda S, Nenoff P, Singal A, Rudramurthy SM, Uhrlass S, et al. The unprecedented epidemic-like scenario of dermatophytosis in India: I. Epidemiology, risk factors and clinical features. Indian J Dermatol Venereol Leprol. 2021;87(2):154-75.
76. Verma SB, Panda S, Nenoff P, Singal A, Rudramurthy SM, Uhrlass S, et al. The unprecedented epidemic-like scenario of dermatophytosis in India: II. Diagnostic methods and taxonomical aspects. Indian J Dermatol Venereol Leprol. 2021;87(4):468-482.
77. Verma SB, Panda S, Nenoff P, Singal A, Rudramurthy SM, Uhrlass S, et al. The unprecedented epidemic-like scenario of dermatophytosis in India: III. Antifungal resistance and treatment options. Indian J Dermatol Venereol Leprol. 20214):468-482.
78. Vollmer RT. Demodex-associated folliculitis. Am J Dermatopathol. 1996;18(6):589-91.

Index

Page numbers followed by *b* refer to box, *f* refer to figure, and *t* refer to table

A

Abrasions 116
Abscesses, subcutaneous 33
Achilles foot project 66
Acne 18
　vulgaris 36
Acquired immunodeficiency
　　syndrome 68, 116, 124
Actinobacteria 4
Adamson's fringe 62
Addison's disease 116, 137
Allylamines 101, 102
Alopecia areata 65
Amorolfine 101, 102, 104
Angular cheilitis 117, 118, 119*f*
Annular erythema 33
Antifungal drugs 106
Antifungal shampoos 108
Aspergillus niger 104
Athlete's foot 36
Atopic dermatitis 16, 17*f*, 65
Atrophic candidiasis
　acute 117, 118
　chronic 117, 118
Aurora borealis pattern 81, 84*f*
Autoimmune polyendocrinopathy
　　candidiasis ectodermal dystrophy
　　126
Azoles 101, 102

B

Bacteria 17*f*
Bacterial flora 5
Bacterial folliculitis 65
Bacterial infections, coexistent 43
Bacterial intertrigo 122
Bacteroidetes 4
Balanoposthitis 117, 120, 121*f*
Barcode-like hairs 83
Beau's lines 72
Bent hair 81*f*, 83, 87
Benzoxaboroles 101, 102
Black dot 83
　tinea capitis 63, 64*f*
Black piedra 138
Borrelia refringens 12
Broken hair 83, 87, 87*f*
Burns 116

C

Cancers 19
　immunology 19
Candida 8, 115, 117, 124
　albicans 14, 67, 74, 94, 115
　dubliniensis 94, 115
　glabrata 94, 115
　infection 116
　krusei 115
　parapsilosis 115
　pseudohyphae 95*f*, 127*f*
　tropicalis 115
Candidal balanitis 117, 120, 121*f*
Candidal balanoposthitis 120*f*
Candidal diaper dermatitis 117, 124
Candidal infections 116, 122, 128
Candidal intertrigo 35, 117, 120, 121*f*,
　　122*f*, 129
　differential diagnosis of 122*b*

Candidal onychomycosis 66, 70, 72, 72f, 128
Candidal paronychia 117, 122, 129
Candidal superinfection 122
Candidal vulvovaginitis 118
Candidiasis 115
  chronic
    hyperplastic 117, 118
    pseudomembranous 117, 118
  congenital 117, 125
  cutaneous 128t
  development of 116t
  diagnosis of 126
  disseminated 117, 124
  perianal 117, 122, 123f
Cavity, oral 116
Cell-mediated immune response 28
Chelates polyvalent metal cations 102
Chemical exposure 137
Chloramphenicol 93
Chronic dermatophytosis 42
  immunopathogenesis of 28
Chronic mucocutaneous candidiasis 117, 125, 130
  autosomal dominant 117, 126
  autosomal recessive 117, 126
  idiopathic 117, 126
Ciclopirox 101, 102, 104
  olamine 102, 103
Circoviruses 9
Clobetasol propionate 24
Clotrimazole 101, 102, 108, 137
Colony-forming units 14
Comma hairs 83
Contraceptives, oral 116
Corkscrew hairs 83
Corticosteroid, signs of 58
Corynebacterium 4
  lipophilicus 6
  minutissimum 6
Coryneform organisms 6
Cosmetics, effects of 14
Cushing's syndrome 116, 131
  iatrogenic 60
Cutaneous candidal infections, clinical manifestations of 117b

Cutibacterium
  acnes 7, 18
  avidum 7
  granulosum 7
Cycloheximide 93

D

Deep folliculitis 35
Demodex
  brevis 9
  folliculorum 9
Denture stomatitis 117, 118
Deoxyribonucleic acid 10
Dermatitis, irritant 43
Dermatophyte 25-27, 66, 67
  scalp infection 61, 79
  septate hyphae 93f
  skin infection 37, 82, 87t
Dermatophytid 40
  management of 40
  reactions 40
Dermatophytoma 85
Dermatophytosis 21, 29, 39f, 99b, 107t
  chronic 42
  diagnosis of 75, 77
  epidemiology of 23
  etiology of 23
  pathogenesis of 25
  recurrent 42
  treatment of 97, 111
Dermatoscopy 77, 79
Dhobi itch 33
Diabetes 116
Diaper candidiasis 117, 124
DiGeorge's syndrome 116
Dimethyl sulfoxide 90
Direct microscopic examination 90
Distal onycholysis 68, 71, 71f
Distal subungual onychomycosis 67, 68, 69f, 85
Double-edged tinea 43
Dried vesicles 87
Drug 102, 106, 107, 111, 112, 128
Dystrophic nails 66

E

Eberconazole 102
Econazole 101, 102, 137
Ectothrix pattern 62
Eczema, chronic 72
Eczematous tinea 43
Edema 120
Efinaconazole 101, 102, 104
Endocrinopathy 117, 126
Endonyx onychomycosis 67, 68, 70*f*, 86
Endothrix pattern 62
Enterococcus faecalis 18
Epidermophyton floccosum 26, 27, 34, 37, 61, 67
Ergosterol synthesis 102
    inhibition of 102, 106
Erythema 55*f*, 83, 87, 121*f*
    diffuse 87
Erythematous candidiasis
    acute 117, 118
    chronic 117, 118
Erythrasma 35, 122, 134
Erythrodermic disease 43
Escherichia coli 7
Excessive sebum production 131
Exophiala werneckii 136
Extensive perifollicular scaling 81*f*
Extensive tinea 46*t*, 47*f*
    corporis 32*f*, 59*f*
    faciei 51*f*
    pseudoimbricata 51*f*

F

Fever, viral 118
Filobasidium floriforme 18
Flexural psoriasis 35, 122
Fluconazole 101, 106-108, 112, 128, 129, 134
    oral 109
Follicular
    flora 18
    inflammatory lesions 50*f*
    keratosis 83

    micropustules 87
Folliculitis decalvans 65
Frontal hair loss 53*f*
Fungal culture 90, 92, 93
Fungal
    flora 8
    infection, cutaneous 87
    invasion 94*f*
Fungi 8
    positive culture for 91*f*
Furunculosis 43

G

Gastrointestinal disturbance 106
Genital candidiasis 129
Genitalia 46*f*
Glabrous skin, tinea of 82
Glucocorticoids 116
Granuloma gluteale infantum 124, 124*f*
Granulomatous disease, chronic 116
Griseofulvin 106-108, 111
    oral 109
Grocott methenamine silver 93
Groins 46*f*, 48*f*

H

Hair 25, 77, 78
    casts 140
Hand, dorsal aspect of 39*f*
Headache 106
Hepatitis 106
Hepatotoxicity 128
Hortaea werneckii 136
Human papilloma virus 9
Human polyomaviruses 9
Hyperkeratosis
    chronic scaly 39*f*
    subungual 68
Hypoadrenalism 126
Hyponychium 68
Hypoparathyroidism 116*t*, 126
Hypothyroidism 116, 126

Index

I

Imidazoles 101
Immune response 26, 27
Immunosuppressives 116
Impetigo 65
Infection
  bacterial 59f
  recalcitrant 107
Inflammation
  absence of 43
  deep-seated 32f
  exaggerated 43
Intense erythema, areas of 87
Intracellular microtubules, inhibition of 106
Intravenous liposomal amphotericin B 128
Invasion, site of 68
Itraconazole 106-108, 112, 128, 134

K

Kerion 65f
Ketoconazole 101, 106, 128, 134, 137

L

Lactation 111, 112
Lactophenol cotton blue mounts 92f
Lateral subungual onychomycosis 67, 68, 69f, 85
Leucyl-tRNA synthetase, inhibition of 102
Leukemia 116
Leukonychia
  acquired 72
  congenital 72
Leukoplakia 118
Lichen planus 58f
Linear erosions over glans 121f
Liver
  disease 111, 112
  function test 112
Luliconazole 102
Lymphomas 116

M

Macrophage function, defective 116
Majocchi granuloma 31
Malassezia 8, 131, 135
  furfur 8, 100
  yeasts 135
Malignancy 116
Malnutrition 131
Merkel cell polyomavirus 9
Methenamine silver stain 127
Miconazole 101, 102, 108, 137
Microbial skin flora 3
Micrococcus
  aggies 6
  kristinae 6
  luteus 6
  lylae 6
  nishinomiyaensis 6
  roseus 6
  sedentarius 6
  varians 6
Microsporum 108
  audouinii 26, 62, 63, 79
  canis 27, 29, 61, 62, 79, 83
  equinum 27, 62
  ferrugineum 26, 62, 63
  fulvum 62
  gallinae 27
  gypseum 26, 62
  incanum 27
  praecox 26
  versicolor 27
Morse code hairs 83, 87
Multiple bent hair 89f
Myalgias 124
Myeloperoxidase deficiency 116
Naftifine 101
Nail 25, 77, 78
  abnormalities 73
  dystrophy, secondary 123f
  fold, inflammation of 122
  infection 74
  lacquers, topical 102
  lichen planus 72
  plate 68, 70f

biopsy 94*f*
brownish discoloration of 72
dorsal surface of 68
invasion of 67
thinning of 72
psoriasis 72
splitting 72
unit, fungal infection of 66

N

Natural killer cells 125
Nausea 106
Neutropenia 124
Neutrophil function, defective 116
Nondermatophyte mould 66-69, 72, 73, 91
  infection 66, 73
Nystatin 101

O

Obesity 116
Oil drop sign 72
Onychocola canadensis 73
Onycholysis 83*f*
  lateral 71
  proximal 68
Onychomycosis 66, 67*t*, 73, 80, 85*t*, 107, 117, 129
  different clinical types of 68*t*
  superficial 67
  total dystrophic 71*f*, 126
  types of 85, 86
Onychoscopy features 85, 86
Oral antifungals 134
  safety profile of 111*t*
Oral candidiasis 116, 117, 129
Oropharyngeal candidiasis 128
Oxiconazole 102

P

Pachyonychia congenita 72
Parasites 9

Paronychia, chronic 123*f*
Patchy hair loss 54*f*
Perifollicular scale 80*f*
Periodic acid-Schiff stain 93, 94*f*, 127
Perioral dermatitis 36
Periungual inflammation 72
Piedra nodules 138, 139*f*
Piedraia hortae 138
Pilar casts 140
Pinta 137
Piroctone olamine 102, 103
Pityriasis
  alba 134
  rosea 33, 134
  rubra pilaris 134
  versicolor 33, 35, 131, 132*f*, 134*t*
    differential diagnosis of 134*b*
Pityrosporum 8
  folliculitis 135*f*
  orbiculare 8
  ovale 8
Polyendocrinopathy 126
Polyenes 101
Polymerase chain reaction 10, 24, 93
Porphyria 106
Porphyromonas gingivalis 12
Posterior scalp, tinea of 54*f*
Potassium hydroxide 54, 90, 93*f*, 133
  mount 57, 62, 95*f*, 127*f*, 133*f*, 136
Potent topical steroids 44
Pregnancy 111, 112, 116
Propionibacterium 4
  acnes 15, 17*f*, 19
Proteobacteria 4
Proximal nail fold 68
  involvement 72
  swelling 72
Proximal nail plate, destruction of 68
Proximal subungual onychomycosis 67, 68, 69*f*, 74, 86
Pruritus 106
Pseudo-leukonychia, patches of 68
Pseudomembranous candidiasis
  acute 116, 117
  oral 117*f*

Psoriasis 17*f*, 18, 33, 65, 134
Psoriatic nails, fungal infection of 71*f*
Pustular tinea 49, 50*f*

R

Recalcitrant dermatophytosis 42, 99
   impact of 60
Red scrotum syndrome 58
Renal disease 111, 112
Rosacea 36

S

Sabouraud's dextrose agar 90, 91, 127, 139
Satellite pustules 122*f*, 123*f*
Scale 83
Scalp
   hair follicles, dermatophytic infection of 61
   skin, superficial dermatophytosis of 43
   tinea of 52, 53*f*
Scaly tinea, diffuse 53
Scopulariopsis brevicaulis 67, 73, 104
Scrotal erythema, persistent 58
Scytalidium dimidiatum 67, 104
Seborrheic dermatitis 10, 18, 33, 35, 65, 122, 134
Selenium sulfide 134
Sertaconazole 102
Serum intracellular adhesion molecules 125
Severe combined immunodeficiency syndrome 116
Skin 25, 77, 78
   dermatophytic infection of 30
   dermatophytosis of 29
   examination of 79
   flora 13, 16, 18
      measurement of 10
      role of 18, 19
   normal flora of 3
   rash 106
   surface biopsy 10

Spaghetti and Meatballs appearance 133*f*
Splinter hemorrhages 72
Squalene epoxidase, inhibition of 102, 106
Staphylococcus
   aureus 6, 13, 16, 35, 118
   capitis 6
   cohnii 6
   epidermidis 6, 19
   haemolyticus 6
   hominis 6
   saccharolyticus 6
   saprophyticus 6
   simulans 6
   warneri 6
   xylosus 6
Steroid
   abuse, signs of 43
   modified tinea 33*f*, 88*f*
   use, chronic 59*f*
Stratum corneum, chronic infection of 131
Striae alba 58
Subacute lupus erythematosus 33
Superficial dermatophytosis 23, 43, 43*b*, 46, 77, 103
   bedside diagnosis of 77
   etiology of 24
Superficial fungal infection 78*t*, 113, 138
Superficial white onychomycosis 68, 70*f*, 86
Sycosis barbae 36
Syphilis 137
   secondary 33, 134
Systemic antifungal 43, 108, 112*t*
   drugs 106*t*
Systemic lupus erythematosus 106
   exacerbation of 106

T

Tannerella forsythia 12
Taste disturbance 106
Tavaborole 101, 102, 105

Index

Telangiectasia 87
Terbinafine 101, 102, 106-108, 111, 112, 134, 137
Therapeutic armamentarium 106
Thiocarbamate antifungals 101
Thrush 117*f*
Thumb nail 69*f*
Thymoma-associated chronic mucocutaneous candidiasis 117, 126
Tinea
  auricularis 43, 51, 53*f*
  barbae 35, 36*f*, 103, 107, 109
    differential diagnosis of 36*b*
  blepharitis 43
  capitis 43, 61, 63*f*, 79, 83*t*, 103, 107, 108
    differential diagnosis of 65, 65*b*
    inflammatory 40, 63, 64*f*
    noninflammatory 63
  corporis 29, 54*f*, 55*f*, 57, 57*f*, 58*f*, 87, 103, 107, 108
    annular lesions of 30*f*
    differential diagnosis of 33*b*
    dumbbell-shaped 43
    extensive truncal 56*f*
    geographic patches of 43
    inflamed lesion of 59*f*, 60*f*
  cruris 23, 33, 34*f*, 48*f*, 87, 103, 107, 108, 122
    differential diagnosis of 35*b*
  faciei 30, 31*f*, 48*f*, 50, 52*f*, 103, 107, 108
    lesion 55*f*
    rising incidence of 43
  genitalis 43
  imbricata 31
  incognito 32, 33*f*, 48, 87
  indecisiva 31, 32*f*
  infections 35, 42, 44, 46, 82*f*, 109, 134
    recalcitrant 46
  labialis 43
  manuum 37, 39*f*, 48*f*, 87, 103, 107, 109
    marginal scale of 87*f*
  nigra 137
    palmaris 136, 137*b*
  pedis 23, 36, 87, 103, 107, 109
    atypical symmetrical 56*f*
    chronic hyperkeratotic 38*f*
    clinical variants of 37*t*
    interdigital 38*f*
    moccasin type of 37
    vesiculobullous type of 37
  pseudoimbricata 43, 48, 49*f*
  unguium 23, 66, 67, 83*f*, 104, 107, 109
    differential diagnosis of 72*t*
  versicolor 131
Tioconazole 101
T-lymphocyte function, defective 116
Tolnaftate 101, 102, 108
Topical antifungal 100, 137
  drugs 100, 102*t*, 105
  shampoos 134
  types of 101*t*
  use of 103
Topical steroid
  abuse 24
  use 55*f*
Translucent hair 88*f*
Treponema
  denticola 12
  macrodentium 12
Triazoles 101
Trichomycosis nodularis 138
  differential diagnosis of 140*b*
Trichophyton 108
  concentricum 26, 61
  equinum 27
  gourville 26
  indotineae 45
  infection, types of 83
  megnini 26, 68
  mentagrophytes 26, 27, 44, 61, 67, 105
  rubrum 24, 26, 29*t*, 37*t*, 44, 67, 68, 104, 105
  syndrome 41, 109, 110*b*

schoenleinii 26, 62, 79
simii 27
soudanense 26, 63, 68
tonsurans 26, 61, 108
verrucosum 27, 62, 67
violaceum 26, 68, 108
yaounde 26
Trichosporon beigelii 138
Trichotillomania 65

U

Ulceration 120
Ultraviolet light 133
Urinary tract infection 8

V

Vaginal candidiasis 117, 118
Vellus hairs 87
  tinea of 43, 57
Viral flora 9

Vitiligo 134
Vulvovaginal candidiasis 117, 118, 119f, 128
  recurrent 128

W

Wavy hair 87
Weight 112
White piedra 138
Wood's lamp 78f, 79
  examination 78, 133

Y

Yeasts 67

Z

Zigzag hairs 83
Zinc pyrithione bar 134
Zoophilic dermatophytes 25

EU GSPR Authorised Reprsentative
Logos Europe, 9 rue Nicolas Poussin
1700, La Rochelle, France
Phone: +33 (0) 6 67 93 73 78
E-mail: contact@logoseurope.eu